PRAISE FOR MIDWIFING MERCY

Vicki Penwell's wonderful book is a powerful reminder that birth is more than a physiological event—it defines a culture, within the setting it occurs, among those who participate in the process and for society as a whole. She thoughtfully conveys this message through grounded examples drawn from her own vast experience and places those events in the larger context of midwifery care throughout the world. The stories she tells provide lessons not just for midwives, but more importantly for all those interested in how we can make birth safer and more humane in these challenging times.

— EUGENE DECLERCQ, PHD – PROFESSOR, BOSTON UNIVERSITY SCHOOL OF PUBLIC HEALTH

Every birth is a threshold, a moment when what we offer a woman either expands or diminishes her sense of what is possible. Midwifing Mercy is Vicki Penwell's nearly fifty-year distillation of what it takes to get that right. It's a book about how culture shapes care, and how care, when it is purposeful and dignified, saves lives.

— NEEL SHAH, MD, OBSTETRICIAN – ASSISTANT PROFESSOR, HARVARD MEDICAL SCHOOL

Vicki Penwell has developed and practiced sustainable models of birth that work to save thousands of lives and bring joy even in the worst of times. She is my cultural hero.

— ROBBIE DAVIS-FLOYD, PHD, MEDICAL ANTHROPOLOGIST – AUTHOR, *BIRTH AS AN AMERICAN RITE OF PASSAGE*

Vicki Penwell has transformed birthing for women and their families the world over. Her career and care is a life-changing commitment to excellence in science and compassion in professional birthing practice.

— ANDRÉ LALONDE, MD, OBSTETRICIAN - ORDER OF CANADA, ADVISOR TO THE WORLD HEALTH ORGANIZATION

As the author of Heart & Hands, the first midwifery textbook for out-of-hospital practice in the United States, I am deeply gratified to see many of the principles of safe and compassionate care that have guided my practice and international teachings for nearly five decades articulated in Vicki's remarkable work. In an era where healthcare is increasingly governed by defensive practices, Vicki teaches sustainability through accountability, care of others through self-care, and how the divinely inspired dedication that has long distinguished the art of midwifery saves lives, heals hearts, and strengthens families. Never has the world needed midwifery more than it does now, and Midwifing Mercy will inspire a new generation to find the humility and the courage to step up to this global health imperative.

— ELIZABETH DAVIS, BA HOLISTIC MATERNITY CARE, CPM

I was brought to tears. Vicki's words hold you, reminding you what it means to feel human again and, more importantly, how to help others feel the same. Through stories of mercy, generosity, and caring for mothers and babies, she beautifully reminds us that healing begins with presence and making people feel seen. This book reconnects us to the humanity that can so easily get lost in a world moving too fast and to the deeper reason so many of us chose this calling in the first place.

— JAMIE J. LIMJOCO, MD, NEONATOLOGIST – ASSOCIATE PROFESSOR, UW SCHOOL OF MEDICINE AND PUBLIC HEALTH

Vicki Penwell has written a rare and necessary book: one that understands that maternal survival, newborn survival, and respectful maternity care are inseparable. Midwifing Mercy is rooted in decades of lived practice and offers a practical, values-driven vision for transforming birth culture through skilled midwifery, evidence-based practice, dignity, compassion, and systems that do not abandon the most vulnerable, or, any women and newborn. For midwives, clinicians, educators, and global health leaders, this is a call to build care that is not only safe, but humane.

— SUELLEN MILLER, PHD, CNM – DIRECTOR OF SAFE MOTHERHOOD PROGRAMS, UCSF

Midwifing Mercy is a transformative and urgently needed contribution to global maternal-child health. Vicki Penwell offers a proven, equity-driven model of midwife-led care rooted in dignity, compassion, radical hospitality, and cultural humility that rebuilds birth culture and saves lives, especially in low-resource settings. This book is a must-read and essential for every midwife and leader committed to building just, community-rooted systems of care.

— TIGIST EJETA, MSN, CPM – PRESIDENT, NATIONAL ASSOCIATION OF CERTIFIED PROFESSIONAL MIDWIVES

Who are the world's most vulnerable people? Without a doubt, pregnant women and newborn babies! In Midwifing Mercy: Reimagining Birth Culture with Strategy and Sacred Purpose, Vicki Penwell documents time-tested, effective strategies to best protect them and urges a call to action to join in this virtuous mission. No one is better qualified to speak, as Vicki Penwell has focused her entire life on serving these precious individuals.

— NICHOLAS COMNINELLIS, MD, MPH – PRESIDENT AND PROFESSOR, INSTITUTE FOR INTERNATIONAL MEDICINE

For almost fifteen years I have been learning from Vicki—and this book feels like a compilation of it all, plus more. From a lifetime of experiences, great depths of wisdom, and hard-won expertise, she inspires, educates, encourages, and challenges midwives to be more merciful, more generous, more excellent, and to never falter in making a difference in the world. Nothing could be more timely.

— ROXANNE ANDERSON, CPM – PRESIDENT, NORTH AMERICAN REGISTRY OF MIDWIVES

Midwifing Mercy is a thoughtful call to transform global birth culture through shared purpose, collaboration, and generosity. Vicki Penwell blends memorable stories with practical wisdom and a clear sense of mission, offering both inspiration and actionable guidance for midwives, birth workers, and those who support them through advocacy and funding. While essential for those committed to respectful and safe maternity care, Midwifing Mercy is also a compelling read for anyone interested in the health and well-being of mothers and babies in our world.

— PAMELA R. DURSO, PHD – PRESIDENT, CENTRAL SEMINARY

Midwifing Mercy offers a heartfelt and visionary guide to transforming maternity care. With wisdom, compassion, and decades of hands-on experience, midwife Vicki Penwell weaves together the why, how, and heart of providing safe, respectful, and purpose-driven care. This book is a must-read for anyone who knows deep within that there is a better, kinder, and more sacred way to bring life into the world, one that empowers MotherBaby-families and fulfills the true calling of midwives and physicians alike.

— DEBRA PASCALI-BONARO, AUTHOR, FILMMAKER – CO-CHAIR, INTERNATIONAL CHILDBIRTH INITIATIVE

This is a brilliant, groundbreaking book. Though it was written for and about birth and midwifery it is far reaching with its sacred concepts that apply to any calling you may have. I am a reader and it is one of the best books I have ever read. Do yourself and your loved ones a favor, read and share this book.

— JAN TRITTEN – FOUNDER OF *MIDWIFERY TODAY* MAGAZINE

Since time immemorial, women have been called to midwifery from a place of purpose and service. As legislation and medicalization have shifted the profession away from its original calling, Vicki Penwell reminds us that midwifing with mercy keeps love at the center—for the midwives who do the work and for the families they care for. In Midwifing Mercy, we are reminded never to lose sight of why we are called to this sacred work.

— SHAFIA MONROE, MPH, DEM, CDT – AUTHOR, *MOTHERING THE MOTHER: AFRICAN AMERICAN POSTPARTUM TRADITIONS, RECIPES, AND HEALING*

MIDWIFING MERCY

REIMAGINING BIRTH CULTURE WITH STRATEGY AND SACRED PURPOSE

VICKI PENWELL

MERCY IN ACTION PRESS

The author receives no personal income from the sale of this book. All proceeds support the charity birth work of Mercy In Action Vineyard, Inc., a 501(c)(3) nonprofit dedicated to improved outcomes in childbirth globally.

Published by Mercy In Action Press

Boise, Idaho, USA

www.midwifingmercy.com

ISBN: 979-8-9953877-0-1

Cover and interior design by Ian Penwell

Disclaimer: This book is intended for informational and educational purposes only. It is not a substitute for professional medical advice, diagnosis, or treatment. Always seek the advice of a qualified healthcare provider with any questions you may have.

Printed in the United States of America

First Edition

To protect the privacy and dignity of the families served, all patient and client names have been changed throughout.

This book is dedicated to Ray Allen, my beloved father, who always told me I was born for a purpose, and to Scott Penwell, my beloved husband, who shared a vocation with me throughout forty-four happy years of marriage. It is impossible to express how much I love and miss them. I am deeply grateful for the gift of being believed in and loved unconditionally by these two extraordinary men.

This book is also dedicated to the next generations of my family, whose love and commitment to mercy and justice give me hope for the future.

CONTENTS

FOREWORD

BY JENNIE JOSEPH

Over a lifetime in this work, I've learned something simple: Some people talk about love, and some people build it into a way of care. There is a kind of care that looks ordinary from the outside, but it changes outcomes because it changes what people believe is possible for them. It changes whether a woman returns for her next visit. Whether she tells the truth about what she's feeling. Whether she calls when something feels wrong. Whether she trusts her own instincts, and whether she trusts you with her fear.

That is why this book matters.

I have known Vicki Penwell long enough to recognize something rare: Her mercy is not a mood. It is a practice. It is structured. It is a discipline. It is a consistent decision to treat women, families, and communities as precious, especially when the world around them has not.

In these pages, you will meet a midwife who does not separate skill from spirit, or excellence from compassion, or outcomes from dignity. You will meet a system builder, someone who has served women and babies in fragile places and then done the harder thing: created a culture that can outlast any one person. That is the kind of leadership our birth world needs more of.

We are living in a moment that lays bare a crisis decades in the making, one in which birth has become, for too many families, a place of fear instead of power, especially for those with the least protection inside the systems around them.

Many people reading this already know that reality intimately. Some have lived it in their own bodies. Some have held the hand of a woman who was not listened to or respected. Some have watched "good care" fail because the environment was rushed, dismissive, or unsafe.

This book answers the question "Is there another way?" not with theory, but with lived, embodied practice.

One of the things I value most about Vicki is that she understands what the modern world keeps trying to train out of us: Authentic relationships are not an "extra." They are not optional. Relationship is protective and strategic.

In my own work, I have always taught that how a person feels in your presence is not incidental; rather, it is part of the intervention. When women feel seen, respected, and safe, they show up differently. Their bodies respond differently. Their families engage differently. Their decisions become clearer. Their courage returns. And care becomes something they can actually receive.

Vicki and I have come to this truth from different roads and different settings, but we recognize each other because the principle is the same: We must build care that restores dignity.

You will see that in her insistence on taking time on purpose.

The world worships efficiency. Healthcare systems are measured by speed and revenue. Schedules are packed. People are processed. And then we act surprised when trust is thin and outcomes suffer.

Vicki challenges that lie with something braver—deliberate human attention. The willingness to "spend" time in the ways that make someone feel protected. The kind of presence that tells a woman without ever needing to say it: *You are not a problem to solve. You are a person to honor.* That kind of care is not sentimental. It is disciplined. It requires leadership. It requires formation, not just training. It requires a culture where everyone from receptionist, student, medical assistant, midwife, and administrator understands that we are not just delivering services, we are shaping an experience of safety.

You will also notice that Vicki is unafraid to speak plainly about character. In a time when people want shortcuts and credentials without cultivation, she reminds us of what seasoned birth workers already know: Who you are shows up in the room. It shows up in an emergency. It shows up when you are tired. It shows up in what you document, what you admit, what you hide, and how you repair. Technique matters and integrity matters too. Accountability matters. Tenderness matters. Truth-telling matters.

And importantly, Vicki does not write from a pedestal. She writes from the field. From the choices that cost something. From the kind of responsibility that forces you back to your purpose again and again. Her faith is not a slogan; it is a source. Whether you share her spiritual language or not, you will recognize its fruit—perseverance, humility, clarity, and a fierce devotion to life.

So what should you expect as you read?

Expect stories that carry both beauty and weight. Expect conviction and practical insight that does not betray the soul of the work. Expect to be challenged, especially if you have accepted what the system calls "normal." And expect to be invited not just to admire what Vicki has built, but to examine what *you* are building in your own corner of birth work.

I am proud to lend my voice here because I trust hers. I trust Vicki's commitment to excellence. I trust her devotion to women and families. I trust the integrity she brings to midwifery. And I trust that anyone who reads this book with an open heart will come away with something we all need right now, renewed courage to practice care that is both merciful and powerful.

May these pages remind you that birth culture can change.

May they remind you that systems can be rebuilt.

May they remind you that your presence matters.

Because that is what a good book should do. It doesn't simply inspire you, it calls you back to the sacred purpose underneath it all.

Jennie Joseph, LM, CPM, RM (UK)
Founder of Commonsense Childbirth
Time Magazine's 2022 Woman of the Year

PREFACE

The baby emerged still and silent, wet, floppy, and breathless on the bed. The young mother looked stricken as she reached out to touch his tiny hand, while the father hovered nearby. Bending low, the midwife calmly whispered a prayer and began the steps of resuscitation. Only two hours earlier, this young couple had been turned away from another medical facility for lack of ability to pay. But they had been welcomed here into Mercy In Action's birth center on this night of labor, and now the air was thick with possibility, suspended between the present reality and an unknown future. When their newborn cried out, it was more than a breath—it was mercy made audible.

Stories like this have a way of touching hearts, challenging the status quo, and shifting cultural beliefs and attitudes. When I started writing this book, I had just completed a dissertation, the final requirement to earn a doctoral degree in creative leadership. I was closing in on fifty years of service in midwifery, both as a practitioner and as an educator. My staff and family had witnessed me writing daily for a year on my dissertation while managing a full workload as the founder and executive director of Mercy In Action, and they encouraged me to keep going and finally start writing the book that tells about our culture and why our methods, strategies, and mindsets have worked so well for so long to improve birth outcomes within our spheres of influence.

This book is my gift to you. If you have picked it up, chances are you care deeply about the health and well-being of mothers and babies in our world. Within these pages, I have gathered the lessons, insights, and earned wisdom that have shaped the work of Mercy In Action over many decades. I share stories of success, setbacks, and innovation, born of both joy and sorrow and always framed with hope for the future.

Think of this as sitting down to share a cup of tea between us while you read each chapter. My hope is that this book becomes a trusted roadmap for midwives, birth workers, and those who support them through advocacy and funding. May it offer inspiration, courage, and clarity, even as it deepens our conviction that birth work is vital and sacred work. I also hope this book offers insight into the joys and challenges faced by those serving on the front lines of maternity care, and awakens a sense of urgency to improve birth outcomes by transforming birth cultures.

I invite you now to journey with me through these pages and discover a vision of what is possible when mercy leads the way and love is the North Star we follow. Step into these stories with a curious mind and an open heart. Put on the kettle, settle in, and let us begin.

INTRODUCTION

All my life, I have been drawn to people who changed their world through lovingly serving those who were poor by earthly standards. Long before I understood my own calling, books became my teachers. Through their pages I began to imagine what a life devoted to meaningful service might look like. These stories shaped my earliest vision for nonprofit work and for a healthcare approach grounded in compassion. The writers who influenced me most were those whose lives reflected the values they taught. Guiding voices such as Mother Teresa, Amy Carmichael, and Jackie Pullinger, along with missionary doctors such as Albert Schweitzer, Thomas Dooley, Dan Fountain, and Paul Farmer, shaped my early understanding that the most faithful strategy begins with walking alongside those who have the least and need our care the most. I was fortunate to later meet or interact with a few of these great humanitarians. I took classes from Dan and Paul, and Jackie became a friend when, for a few years, we sent teams back and forth between Hong Kong and the Philippines.

In 1980, I began training to be a midwife, and the seeds were planted for what would become Mercy In Action, the global nonprofit I founded with my late husband, Scott. The methods and strategies in this book emerge from a lifetime lived at the intersection of health-care, cross-cultural service, and a deep commitment to mercy and compassion. My vocation has taken me from Arctic Alaska to the rainforest coastlines of the Philippines; from inner-city communities in Mexico and Cambodia to international conference stages in Europe and the United States; and from steep Himalayan trails in India and Nepal to equally steep learning curves in seminary, studying adaptive challenges and design theory. I have worked along-side an exceptional community of colleagues and students whose insight, energy, and passion have inspired me. Every day I count myself fortunate to get to do this work.

Through it all, I have come to believe this truth with my whole heart: The way we approach birth is not just about a biological event. Instead, birth is a sacred threshold that holds up a mirror to how well we value life. Alarmingly, maternity care seems to be in crisis throughout most of the world, as maternal and neonatal mortality rates continue to be unacceptably high. More than any other measur-able health indicator, these statistics reveal the great divide between rich and poor. Maternity care is also the area within healthcare where patient abuse is most prevalent and human rights are least protected, according to researchers.

This book reflects my commitment to embodying a culture of sharing knowledge. In Part One, we will explore a transformative worldview, delving into the motivation, inspiration, and sense of purpose that fuel our calling. We will examine character traits that affect birth outcomes, and we will reflect on hospitality and the concept of servant leadership. In Part Two, I will share the practical frameworks and birth models that have shaped our global impact, and disclose our inventions, innovations, and unique mindsets used to achieve these outcomes. In Part Three, we'll look outward together, exploring how generosity and global collaboration can transform maternity care worldwide, leading to better outcomes even in the most difficult circumstances. We will explore what it looks like to work in contexts of disaster and poverty, and how to continue as a lifelong learner. To help paint pictures in the minds of my readers, I have interspersed many stories among the descriptions of our model—tales of mercy, practiced over decades in the messy, miraculous context of real life.

A few years ago, we were invited to share our results with a large and well-known global foundation examining the impact of midwifery funding on maternal and infant survival rates. The person presenting on our behalf was allotted time to present only two slides. So Nicole Werner, a graduate of our College of Midwifery who has a PhD and volunteers her research expertise to analyze and compile our data, created graphics that convey the statistical outcomes from our Philippine birth centers.

- Mercy In Action (a United States-based 501(c)(3) nonprofit) has built and supported birth centers in the Philippines since 1991. Funding only midwife-led facilities that use the Midwives Model of Care© and follow the International Childbirth Initiative (ICI) 12 Steps to Safe and Respectful MotherBaby-Family Maternity Care, Mercy In Action has served over 17,000 families while keeping detailed statistics.
- By applying evidence-based practices, we have demonstrated that all complications are low and maternal and neonatal deaths remain well below national rates, even in the face of numerous systemic risk factors in our served population (e.g., chronic malnutrition, low socioeconomic standing).
- Patient satisfaction based on women's questionnaires is consistently high.

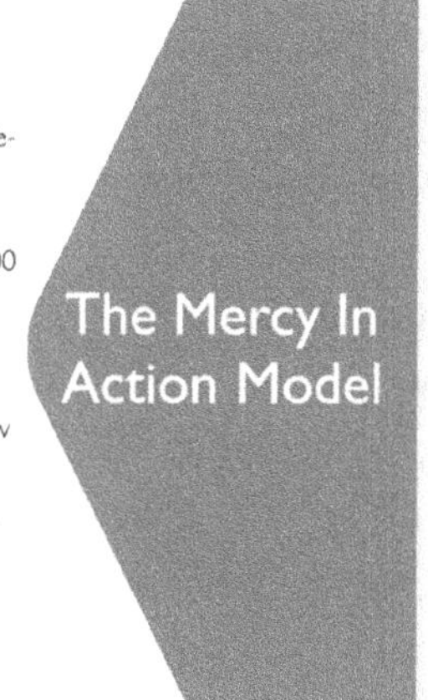

This book contains our secrets to achieving these incredible outcomes. Each chapter is grounded in practical strategies that have been lived, tested, and proven over decades of service and thousands of births in our settings where this data was collected. Through Mercy In Action, we have built something quietly revolutionary: a midwife-led, compassion-fueled system of maternal and newborn care that treats every person with dignity and removes barriers to lifesaving care, with documented outcomes that would be impressive anywhere.

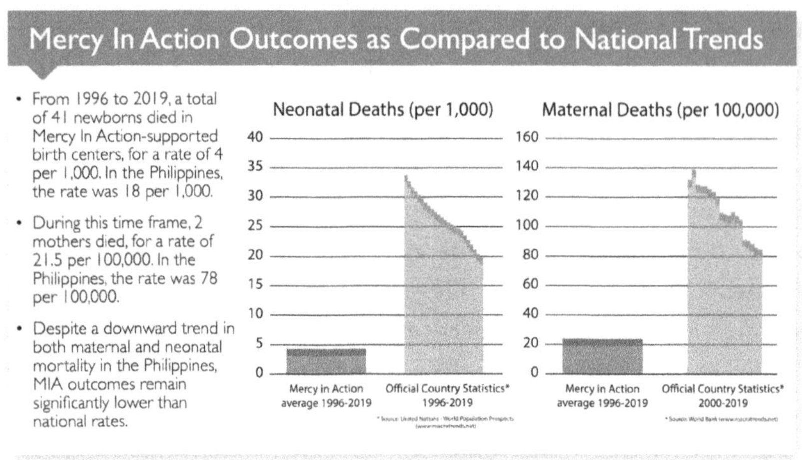

While you will not find clinical midwifery skills taught in this book, you will find plenty of practical "soft skills" necessary to serve well and be the best midwife or birth worker you can be. It is about an orientation of the mind, a directional compass to guide our day-to-day choices, the attitudes and thinking patterns we can learn to adopt, and the myriad ways we can open our hearts a bit wider. Once you recognize the shifts required to transform birth culture, some subtle and others seismic, you will see powerful hints in every chapter pointing to how our sustained vision over decades has indeed changed birth culture.

Scholars in sociology and anthropology commonly define culture as a set of shared beliefs, values, attitudes, standards, and behaviors. That definition, while correct, still falls short. Any organization's cultural expression is ultimately about how we treat one another. What people say they believe or value isn't as important as what they do. No amount of brilliantly worded mission statements or cozily decorated delivery rooms can make up for a genuine culture where birth is safe and mothers, babies, and their families are treated with respect. When we center our culture around treating people right, everything else will eventually fall into place.

One more thing: Words can be a source of connection or misunderstanding, as I know well from living in multiple countries, cultures, customs, and dialects throughout my life. The choice of wording used in this book is intended for a global audience, with respect to those who choose to use different language around the subject matter of birth.

PART I

A CULTURE OF SERVING WITH PURPOSE

EMBRACING THE CALL TO MAKE A DIFFERENCE

A Tale of Prenatal Outreach: Myrna's Story

This story is based on the experience of a woman encountered in a recovering disaster zone in the Philippines where Mercy In Action supports a local birth center.

Myrna lived at the edge of a shattered world. Her small shack sat on the outskirts of a coastal village still clawing its way back from the devastation of a typhoon that had ripped through two years earlier. Uprooted trees leaned like weary sentinels, and the remains of broken houses stood as hollow reminders of what once was. Her own home was a fragile shelter pieced together from scraps of lumber, warped plywood, and bits of tin pulled from the rubble. When the storm came, it took her parents and everything they owned. What it left behind was her determination to survive.

By the time her pregnancy began to show, Myrna was already bone-weary from survival. Each morning, she swept the dirt floor of her shack, trying to impose order on the chaos around her. For meals, she cooked rice over a small charcoal stove, the smoke stinging her eyes as she fanned the flame to life. When her new husband was lucky enough to find day labor work, they would sometimes add small bits of organ meat or fish to the meager vegetables she grew. Nights were long and colored by worry, as wind rattled the loose metal roof, and memories of that storm replayed in her mind. She missed her mother most when the baby kicked.

Myrna did not know if any clinics would accept her into care; she could not afford the fees required for a pregnancy checkup. Still, she prayed quietly every night for her baby to be born healthy.

One morning in her eighth month, while sorting through a pile of used plastic bottles to sell, Myrna overheard two neighbor women talking. "They say there's a party for pregnant women next week at the barangay center," one of them said. "Free food, maybe even free checkups."

Myrna froze. The idea sounded impossible. Free care had dried up after the disaster responders left the island. She had learned from expe-

rience to be wary of promises. But something in her heart stirred. On her way home she walked past the community center and saw the poster advertising an upcoming buntis party. That night, as the kerosene lamp flickered and her baby rolled inside her, she lay awake listening to the rain tap against her tin roof, wondering if she dared believe it.

On the morning of the event, Myrna woke before dawn. She washed her face in cold water, combed her hair, and put on her cleanest dress, faded blue cotton with patches on one sleeve. Her stomach fluttered from nerves as she walked the long dusty road toward the barangay hall.

When she arrived, she hesitated at the entrance, expecting someone to ask for payment. No one did. Instead, smiling faces greeted her. A young woman handed her a cup of water and led her to a seat in the shade. Another smiling woman who identified herself as a midwife took her hand and said, "Welcome." Myrna looked around and realized she was seated among other women with round bellies like hers, as well as a few men and older women who were there as companions. Preschool-age children played around the edges of the group, darting in and out.

Then the main event began with a prayer and greetings from a local health official. Two midwives introduced themselves and began a health lesson, holding up bright posters. Myrna listened while the midwives spoke about caring for the baby growing inside her, about nutrition, rest, and prenatal care. They introduced the First 1,000 Days program, explaining how it supports her baby's development from pregnancy through two years of age. They shared their commitment to keeping birth gentle and respectful for every mother. The midwives' voices were kind. They laughed easily. For the first time in months, she felt like she wasn't holding her breath anymore.

When the teaching ended, someone pressed a small bottle of prenatal vitamins into her palm. She stared at it in disbelief, the way one might look at a handful of jewels. Later, trays of food appeared: a hot meal of rice, vegetables, and chicken. Myrna ate slowly, almost reverently, as though she might wake and find it had been a dream.

Then, to her astonishment, all the pregnant women in attendance were called to the front, and she was handed a small gift packet containing items needed for a new baby, including a bar of soap and a soft baby hat. Tears filled her eyes as she held the little hat against her cheek.

As she was leaving, one of the midwives leaned close and hugged her, saying, "Our birth center is nearby. You can come for prenatal care. You can give birth there with your husband beside you when the time comes. There is no fee to you or your family."

For a moment, Myrna could not speak. She could only nod, her throat tight with emotion. She walked home in the late afternoon light, clutching the vitamins and gift packet to her chest, her steps lighter than they had been in a while. For the first time since the typhoon, hope had found her, and the hope felt big enough to encompass her soon-to-be-born baby.

Myrna went to the clinic for a prenatal checkup. She was amazed to find the midwives remembered her name. She returned when contractions began, and they monitored her labor, showing her husband how to rub her aching back, whispering encouragement as the hours passed. Myrna felt safe and gave in to the waves of contraction pain that washed over her. When her baby girl's first cry filled the room, Myrna reached out with joy and knew with certainty that the future was no longer something to fear.

1
BEGIN WITH WHY

I don't know what your destiny will be, but one thing I know: The only ones among you who will be really happy are those who will have sought and found how to serve.

— ALBERT SCHWEITZER

BEFORE WE BEGIN TO TALK ABOUT WHAT WE DO IN BIRTH WORK, OR HOW we do it, we must start with *why* we do it. Why begin with *why*? Our *why* is the beating heart of everything that follows; it gives our lives the purpose we need to sustain this service profession we signed up for. Our *why*, if we keep it front and center, becomes our daily motivation. It has the power to define our sacred purpose. The ability to express our *why* also invites friends and loved ones to better support us once they understand the deeper purpose behind the unconventional life we have chosen. Support has been proven in recent studies to be essential to a midwife's wellbeing, which is why sharing our purpose in an effective manner could help clarify our mission and mitigate burnout among healthcare workers.

PEOPLE BUY WHY

"People don't buy *what* you do; they buy *why* you *do* it." Simon Sinek uses these words to inspire leaders, and he is convinced from his work studying business that any great venture starts with being able to articulate why the venture exists. Probably anyone can explain what they do, and some can explain how they do it, but very few can clearly explain why they do what they do. Yet the why is the very thing, if the cause is noble, that inspires us and those around us to do the hard work necessary to create, launch, and sustain good work. Without a clearly articulated why, leaders and their followers flounder, and the public never understands the mission, no matter how honorable it may have seemed to the founders.

Our mission will only carry us as far as our meaning goes. If we are going to live a purposeful life and motivate ourselves to persist when it gets hard, we must keep returning to our why. And if we are going to inspire anyone else along the way to join us in taking action, why we do what we do, as well as what we do, must resonate with them. Starting with why is a secret to successful strategic midwifery.

I am fascinated by people who look at the world differently and who can articulate what they see. In my life, I have sought to stay curious and take a creative and open approach to everything life throws at me. Starting with *why* is a powerful way of looking at our work differently. In the past few years I have been more deliberate about how I communicate with people on my team and in the broader world. I consciously try to always start with why, rather than what or how, for anything I am explaining. This changes the conversation, whether it is a new idea or ensuring that our decades-long mission continues in the same direction.

Making this change in how I frame things has brought new awareness to me of how often we default to talking about *what* first, maybe because that is often the thing people ask: "What do you do?" We could answer with the *what*, and usually do; after all, that was the question. So I may say, "I am a midwife, I work for a nonprofit, I live in Asia and support accessible maternity care, I founded a midwifery college," etc.

Since most of us in birth work like to take action—we are givers and doers—we may also spend time talking about the *how* of what we do: how we provide support, how we advocate, how we protect natural birth. We may even talk about the *where* of what we do, like working in a hospital, birth center, or at home births.

The trouble is, when someone asks us what we do, the conversation may end before we ever get around to speaking about the most interesting, if not the most important, things to know about each of us. If you don't share your *why*, people who meet you will never truly know you. And you may not truly know yourself. If you have misplaced or forgotten your why, could it be that you never really focused on the reasons you were doing what you do in the first place?

WHY MAKES MEANING

As wonderful as it is to be a giver and a doer, as most health workers are, we are the people most in danger of burnout. Without anchoring ourselves in the deep reasons behind why we do this work, we will always be at risk of growing weary and quitting. Tragically, some midwives who started with loads of zeal and compassion become cynical and jaded as the years go by. This is sometimes a result of losing focus on the goal and losing sight of our meaning and purpose. Of course, burnout has also been linked to many other causes, such as lack of time off or cumulative traumatic stress. It could be due to lacking a healthy perspective or lacking enough support. Regardless, having a driving purpose in life will motivate us to find a way through problems we encounter along the way.

Action without purpose can't sustain us. Passion for birth work may burn hot and fast, but purpose is what carries us forward and will make our work sustainable in the long run. Our why is our life's purpose, and our life's purpose should be our why. Why is what gives our work the meaning we need to do this job well and find joy in the journey.

Knowing our why doesn't just give us direction; it helps build resilience. It roots us and grounds us when the suffering and fatigue we encounter in pursuit of our calling become overwhelming at times. Our why reminds us that what we do matters, and that doing it with excellence matters too, even when no one sees it or appreciates our sacrifices. Without a strong purposeful sense of why, we may eventually become overwhelmed by the responsibility, if not the sheer exhaustion, involved in long-term birth work. This is a great loss not just for the individual midwife who burns out, but for the entire community that is no longer served.

WHY IS PERSONAL

Our why is going to be deeply personal to each of us. The foundation for my own life's work as a midwife, educator, and nonprofit founder is the belief I hold that God is loving and merciful beyond all reason, and human beings are precious because we are created in the image of God. I believe it is an injustice that some mothers and babies are not valued and cared for the way they deserve to be, causing their pregnancy journey to end with suffering and loss rather than resulting in healthy new life. The world I envision is a world where no mother or baby suffers harm needlessly or dies in childbirth from preventable causes. That belief and vision has shaped everything about my life's work for almost fifty years and turned it into a vocation rather than a career.

EACH BIRTH MATTERS

One story that captures the heart of my why took place in 2006 when we were living in a remote village on Mindoro Island in the Philippines. Before dawn, our staff midwife and I climbed into a *tricy*, a small motorcycle with a sidecar, along with two midwifery students. We rattled up a rutted dirt road toward the sea, the early morning air still heavy with salt and mist.

Amihan lived with her husband and eight children in a small two-room bamboo and plywood home. The house had no glass or screens on the windows and no indoor plumbing, and the rough-hewn furnishings were simple and utilitarian. When we arrived, Amihan was already in the transition stage of labor, lying on her side on a bare wooden bed. We sat quietly beside her, monitoring vital signs but otherwise not disturbing her. I remember listening to the sound of waves breaking against the shore below and thinking they seemed in rhythm with her contractions.

Delivering a ninth baby carries real risk, but this time she was not alone. Amihan had birthed all eight of her previous children without a trained birth attendant present, because like many women worldwide, she had no money to spend on healthcare. But that morning was different. She gave birth to a healthy baby girl, attended with loving care by two trained and equipped midwives, and her excessive bleeding after the birth was quickly stopped by skilled hands. Being there beside Amihan as her bleeding slowed and her strength returned, I was struck by how thin the line is between life and death for so many mothers, and how unnecessary that line often is. What saved her was not advanced technology or being in a hospital, but the presence of skilled midwives who knew what to do and acted without delay. The thankfulness she expressed over and over for our coming to her humble home that day reminded me again why midwives matter so deeply.

This is why my work is devoted to supporting and funding midwives and midwife education around the world: so that no woman gives birth without skilled care simply because of where she lives or what she can afford. Helping to ensure that women everywhere have access to trained midwives when they need them most is a driving purpose of my life.

The next day when I arrived at Amihan's house on the back of my husband's motorcycle for her twenty-four-hour postpartum checkup, she met us at the door with a big smile. Cradling her newborn, she told Scott she could not believe how cared-for she felt. As I checked the baby's cord and reiterated how to prevent infection, we discussed the usual feeding practices in her community, and I encouraged her to continue breastfeeding exclusively for the first six months. We parted with a hug, and I told her someone on our midwifery team would return for several more visits in the following weeks.

Simple steps like these—skilled attendance at birth in any setting, clean cord care of the newborn, and exclusive breastfeeding—save millions of lives every year. We know that. Yet millions of families still face birth without skilled, safe, and respectful help. That reality continues to shape my purpose and fuels my why.

WHEN WE FORGET WHY

At times over the decades, I have temporarily forgotten that I am choosing to live my life within a vocational framework, and discouragement has followed. Purpose does not sustain itself without care. It must be remembered and renewed. When I lose sight of this, I need moments of honest reckoning that draw me back to first principles. Within the Judeo-Christian tradition that has shaped me, the greatest commandment is to love God with all our heart, soul, mind, and strength, and to love our neighbor as ourselves. This way of life calls for mercy, justice, compassion, and relationship, not as abstract ideals, but as lived commitment.

Rekindling my *why* often begins with returning to these foundations in tangible ways. I reread the lives of those who have walked a similar path before me with courage and humility—little-known heroes like Father Damien of Molokai, whose faith expressed itself through presence among the suffering. Stories like his remind me that sustained purpose is built through small acts of love repeated over time. I listen more carefully to the stories of those I serve. I pray, asking for my heart to be reoriented to the way Jesus treated people when He walked the earth. I seek out others who are living their own callings with integrity, allowing their witness to strengthen my own resolve. In remembering the big picture, I return to my purpose, and my personal why is made clear again.

I founded Mercy In Action Vineyard, Inc. and before that, Via Vita Health Project, Inc., as nonprofit organizations dedicated to promoting safe birth, because I believe that everyone deserves to survive childbirth. I believe that all children deserve to be valued simply because human beings are of infinite worth. The love of God compels me to spend my life finding ways to build and fund birth centers and clinics that are committed to excellence for people living in poverty. The need for more well-trained midwives around the world compels me to teach and inspire the next generation of midwives to meet the urgent needs of their own communities all over the world. Doing this through a nonprofit framework has allowed me to share the joy of serving every day with dozens of like-minded co-laborers and thousands of good-hearted supporters and donors, which further reinforces my personal why.

At its core, my personal and professional vocation boils down to loving God and people. It is what gets me out of bed each morning and gives my life meaning. I wake up and ask myself, "Who is my neighbor today?" Thus, as Gene Edward Veith says in his book on vocation, the ultimate test of whether we are being called to something is to ask, "How does my calling serve my neighbor?"

You may not be coming from the same spiritual place I am, but the principle is the same: Begin with discovering your personal why, whatever that looks like to you. We all need a sense of sacred purpose in life, whether or not it is tied to any particular faith tradition. Within birth work, that sacred purpose is often expressed as our lives being devoted to a service that we regard as highly important, meaningful, and worthy of our very best effort.

THE CRISIS BEFORE US

A quiet crisis is happening every day in our world. It is a crisis that rarely makes headlines but relentlessly continues to steal lives. It happens during birth, in those fragile hours surrounding the arrival of new life. Too many women wonder if labor contractions will trap them in a nightmare of obstructed labor, ending in a fistula or death, or if they will survive delivery only to succumb in the early postpartum days to infection, hemorrhage, or hypertensive disorders.

The crisis in the way maternal and child healthcare is given and received is hardly an abstract thought for those of us who live and work in the world's most vulnerable communities. It is a daily reality.

At the time of this publication, every day approximately seven hundred women die in childbirth in the world, which works out to one death every two minutes, from one of those four medical causes I just listed. That is akin to a passenger plane crashing several times a day. And that's just the mothers. More than six thousand newborns die every single day in their vulnerable first four weeks after birth. Two million more babies are stillborn each year.

The vast majority of these deaths are preventable, which is what makes it so tragic and unjust. The root causes appear to be poverty, neglect, abuse, and sometimes, the overuse of medical technology.

The Philippines, my adopted "other home" since 1991, is among fifty-eight countries the United Nations has identified as not being on track to reach the Sustainable Development Goals for maternal and child health. The majority of maternal and newborn deaths still occur in these less-developed countries. In the Philippines, as in many parts of the world, it is common for families to brace for the worst during childbirth, fearing that the baby may not survive, and knowing the mother's life is at risk as well. As a midwife, I often see both surprise and relief on the family's faces when their newborn arrives safely. This heartbreaking expectancy of loss is reflected in the way many couples delay naming their babies, aware as they are of the stark reality that newborns in their settings are often stillborn or die shortly after birth.

Regardless of a country's ranking on the survival list, it is the poor, the marginalized, and the voiceless who bear the heaviest burden, even in richer nations. Mothers and babies from low socioeconomic communities, tribal and ethnic minorities, or any group discriminated against often suffer disproportionately. Within a single country, access to respectful and safe maternity care can vary dramatically depending on where you live and what you can afford to pay.

Behind every statistic are real flesh-and-blood people. A mother who labors alone with no trained help. A baby who dies within hours of being born because there was no clean, safe place to arrive into the world. A maternity care system built around caring for those who have good insurance. A family forced deeper into poverty by medical bills they can never pay.

In parts of the world where the risk of dying in childbirth is high, it's not uncommon for a mother to say goodbye to her other children as labor begins. "I am going now to get a new baby for the family," she tells them, "but it is a long and dangerous journey, and I may not return."

And it's not just about medical safety. Around the world, women labor under harsh conditions in overcrowded hospitals or ill-prepared homes. In the latter, they may be subjected to what has been called "deadly neglect." Ignored and undervalued, they are perhaps sent to the cowshed to deliver because the blood involved in birth makes them unclean. In the former, what is referred to as "obstetric violence" has been identified in many health facilities, where women are routinely shouted at, slapped, denied the presence of a loved one, and subjected to non-evidence-based medical interventions that leave them traumatized in body and soul. Babies are often taken away to another room after birth and not returned for hours, despite their greatest need being what only their own mother can provide.

IT SHOULD BE NORMAL FOR NOBODY

A missionary who had served in Malawi told a story about mentioning to an acquaintance there that she was grieving the loss of a friend's baby back in America. The Malawian woman replied simply, "Unusual for you Americans. Normal for us."

These soul-crushing realities are the backdrop to everything I do. From personal experience, I know these are not just numbers; they are lives cut short and futures stolen, often for lack of access to respectful, skilled, and compassionate care. This is the "normal" we refuse to accept within my organization, Mercy In Action. The world may call it inevitable, but we believe it's changeable.

Almost 95% of all global maternal deaths occur in low-income and lower-middle-income countries. The vast majority are concentrated in the regions of sub-Saharan Africa and South Asia, and experts say most of these deaths could be prevented. In contrast, countries like Norway and the Netherlands have some of the lowest maternal mortality rates in the world, thanks in part to their robust integration of midwifery services throughout pregnancy, birth, and the postpartum period. Their health systems center on high-quality, accessible, and affordable midwife-led care, emphasizing natural, physiological birth. High-risk pregnancy is identified early, allowing for specialized, higher-level care, yet these countries have a relatively low cesarean section rate.

The United States falls somewhere between these two extremes, with one of the highest maternal mortality rates among industrialized countries. It is important to note that maternal mortality captures only the worst outcome; what is not reflected in mortality rates is how many women suffer greatly and come close to dying. The World Health Organization defines a "maternal near miss" as a woman who nearly died but survived a life-threatening complication during pregnancy, childbirth, or shortly afterward. Near misses are far more common than deaths and indicate moments when care may have been delayed or systems failed.

Near misses are sometimes framed as "successes," but more accurately, they are signals of serious breakdowns in care that should largely be preventable. No one who enters a hospital healthy to have a baby should expect to leave through an intensive care unit, or to have long-term negative effects of barely surviving. Near-miss data reveals an uncomfortable truth about how often childbirth becomes unnecessarily dangerous, even when death is avoided.

Since we know what is possible, we must do better for every mother, every baby, and every community still waiting to survive childbirth without tragedy. Our deepest reason for being midwives means we must refuse to let these mortalities and morbidities be dismissed as routine. We must refuse to let despair write the final chapter. This is where our work begins. Let's work toward every country being a safe place to give birth. Let's create a solid strategy based on love and service, to see things turn around in our lifetime, everywhere we have influence.

THE POWER OF WHY

In the face of such staggering need, it would be easy to give in to despair, but purpose has the power to cut through despair. Purpose emerges when we start each day with a clear understanding of our why. It is how the vision remains intact, one day at a time, as the years slide by. Without a clear sense of purpose, we can lose our way.

I began serving women and babies through midwifery at the tender age of twenty-one years old. I quickly formed a deep conviction that no one should suffer harm or die during pregnancy or childbirth due to neglect or preventable causes. Since 1980, midwifery has been more than a career for me. It's been a calling, and I have felt it my life's vocation to restore value to those who are not valued by the world.

It has not always been an easy life. There are a thousand different ways this work can break your heart. Along with all the beautiful births, I have also visited pregnant inmates in prison, midwifed births in a tent for traumatized survivors of natural disaster, and listened to the raw, primal wails of grieving families. The circumstances may vary, but my response to both joy and suffering around childbirth is rooted in something that remains constant: Every mother, every baby, every family deserves to be treated with the utmost dignity and the most excellent care around the time of pregnancy and childbirth.

THE VALUE OF ONE

This conviction that each life has value runs deep in our shared work with our Mercy In Action teams. It's what led Marlene, one of our midwife directors in the Philippines, to suggest an unusual name for our newest project: Imago Dei Health & Birth Center. *Imago Dei* is a Latin phrase meaning "image of God," and she couldn't get it out of her mind as we began planning this new birth center a few years ago. She said the name came to her again and again, while daydreaming about the center, lying awake at night, even standing in the shower. It just kept surfacing, as if it had already chosen us. Marlene's background lends particular weight to her connection with this idea. She gave me permission to share parts of her story here, to show why questions of worth have shaped her so profoundly.

A DIFFICULT PAST

Marlene grew up feeling anything but valued. She was aware from her earliest memory that she had been abandoned as a baby, left for someone to find. She was often labeled a "foundling" as she grew up in Manila, a title she experienced as derogatory. Doomed to go through life without the love and protection of parents, at a young age she ended up on the streets, which quickly led to the downward spiral of petty crime, drugs, and selling her body simply to survive. It meant beatings and danger and occasional time behind bars. Her whole life had been undervalued from the very start; she was, by her own description, what people think of as a throwaway of society. Aware that people who saw her on the street passed judgment, she experienced shame for things beyond her control. Often hungry and scared, sometimes hurt and alone, Marlene was treated with contempt but rarely pity. Her life was as inevitable as it was unenviable.

One day, she had a chance encounter with another prostitute who had left the streets and said a profound spiritual experience had led her to seek help. Shortly thereafter, she met a group of missionaries from different Asian nations and remembers being told for the first time that she was created in the image of God. Amazed by this news, she was still reluctant to trust, until the day, as Marlene tells it, she had her own powerful encounter with God.

"I saw a woman, around fifty years old, still working on the street, and a question suddenly hit me: 'Is this really the life you want?' That moment broke something in me. I cried out to God and prayed, 'I'm tired. I want to leave the streets, but I don't know how. Please help me.' The very next day, Ate G came and brought me to Olongapo."

With only a mustard-seed-sized faith at first, Marlene dared believe that another life was possible for her and she was worthy of something better. She entered a live-in rehabilitation program for sexually exploited women. After a year there, she was offered the opportunity to attend midwifery school on a scholarship. Upon her graduation in 2012, the director of her program approached me about giving Marlene a job, and that is how we met.

Marlene's value and worth were of course there all along; she just did not know it. Today, when you walk into our Olongapo clinic, Marlene greets you with a beaming smile and a welcome that makes you feel instantly at home. Spend a little time with her, and you will be impressed by her kind, loving, and outgoing demeanor. You would probably also notice her bright, inquisitive mind, her sense of humor, and her radiant joy. And if you were lucky enough to know her well, as I do, you would realize she is also a fiercely loyal and trustworthy friend.

Marlene discovered the words *imago Dei* when she enrolled in Bible school after finishing midwifery school, but she had discovered the concept when still living on the street. Marlene found self-worth and a vision for how she wants to lift other downtrodden women. Devoting her days and boundless energy to giving care, respect, and a sense of value to women who have rarely received it, Marlene has found her why.

INHERENT WORTH

Within the belief system of the faith Marlene and I share, it is not an option to ignore the needs of the poor or retain the right to discriminate against anyone. *Imago Dei* is a concept that turns strangers into family. Whether you use this specific language or use a non-religious framing, the concept is simple: Every person carries value that can't be measured by social status, income, education, or any other metrics. When local people ask about the name of our clinic and we explain the meaning of *imago Dei* to them, something often shifts visibly in their demeanor: Their shoulders straighten, their eyes light up, and they walk away not just informed, but affirmed. Maybe it's the first time they've heard that they are worthy, that they belong with dignity in the family of humankind.

ANTIDOTE FOR BURNOUT

When our work is anchored in the clarity of purpose, midwifery becomes more than just a profession or a service. It becomes a reflection of our values, our humanity, and our hope. And that can make the difference in our "expiration date" as midwives!

Those of us who give and give, from the deep places in our hearts, are especially at risk for deep fatigue, maybe even burnout, unless we stay connected to our deeper purpose. Generosity on its own can wear thin. But generosity rooted in meaning, and tied to a sense of sacred purpose, can last.

Birth work is often demanding—physically, emotionally, and spiritually. It is when we stay rooted in our purpose that even the most difficult days begin to make sense. It is only when we know and remember our why, when we're anchored in compassion, hope, and optimism, that the outcomes begin to shift. With a sense of purpose, we become the kind of midwives who do everything with excellence, and that can't help but be reflected in our care and in our outcomes. As you become clear about your underlying purpose, weariness can begin to ease, allowing you to step back and see the bigger picture of your calling.

CALLING

For me, this calling has always been both practical and deeply personal. I've spent decades walking alongside mothers and babies in places where birth can be as dangerous as it is beautiful. From the beginning, when my husband and I started our first nonprofit organization to build, fund, and staff birth centers in areas where access to safe care was limited or nonexistent, our commitment has been to offer excellence, not just access; mercy, not just midwifery.

Over the years, I've had the privilege of taking part in the training of thousands of midwives, doctors, community health workers, doulas, and childbirth educators from around the world. Each year, our teaching faculty welcomes around fifty new students into our accredited college of midwifery. We teach continuing education courses to hundreds of midwives each year around the world, both live and online. All of them are learners who bring their own passion and purpose to this sacred calling. Through every lesson taught, every story shared, and every life touched, we have returned again and again to one guiding question: How can we make birth safer, more respectful, and more just? And how can we extend that kind of care to everyone who longs for it but may not have access?

SACRED PURPOSE

Along the way, I've discovered something important. Transformation of birth culture doesn't come through complaining about what is wrong. Though it is understandable to fall into criticism and blaming, it is rarely helpful and may lead us to despair. No, the change the world needs comes through acts of love and service, and through being diligent to keep the vision of what birth could be. Transformation comes when we tap into divine love, when we serve, when we listen and bear witness to the stories, when we let ourselves be changed.

That's what we mean when we talk about sacred purpose. It doesn't always feel dramatic and it doesn't need to draw attention, but it anchors us in meaning. It reminds us that our work is not just about monitoring pregnancy and caring for babies. It's about standing in the gap between death and life, fear and trust, vulnerability and strength. We do this with an equal mix of compassion and skill so that all births for all people at all times are both safe and respectful.

FINDING MERCY

Once, a woman who lived on the edge of the city dump discovered she was expecting a baby. Her name was Dalisay. Each day she picked her way across the smoking piles of garbage, searching for anything of value she could sell. The air was thick with the acrid smell of burning plastic and rotting food, and the trash heaps often smoldered from spontaneous combustion. Dalisay tried to ignore her pregnancy for as long as she could. She had no money to pay for a checkup, and fear pressed down on her as heavily as the heat.

One day, while scavenging through the landfill, she overheard a neighbor mention a place that offered free prenatal care. She could hardly believe such a place existed, and only one barangay (district) away. She was certain if it did exist, they would never accept someone who lived among the garbage. Weeks passed before she gathered the courage to try.

At last, with her belly growing and no other options, Dalisay set out to find the clinic. She walked for miles, following directions she had pieced together from bits of rumor. When she reached the neighborhood, nothing looked familiar, and she soon realized she was lost. In her desperation, she began stopping strangers to ask if they knew where the free maternity clinic could be found. When she finally arrived at our clinic and rang the bell, I opened the door and invited her in, and she said these words: "I have been asking everyone, everywhere...where can I find Mercy?"

She was, of course, referring to Mercy In Action, the clinic. But in that moment, I knew she was also asking a bigger, existential question, one that so many people carry, often without words: "Where can I find mercy? Where can I go to be seen with compassion? Where can I feel safe? Who will meet me in my vulnerability and not turn me away for lack of money to pay?"

Dalisay was searching that day not just for a building, but for something deeper. That question, that cry for mercy, is one we've heard echoed again and again in our work. Several of our team members have told me that they have heard these exact same words, "I was searching for Mercy," or "I was looking everywhere for Mercy," when a woman arrives at our clinic doors, reflecting the fact that our name is often abbreviated by the local people. Still, it is a powerful image.

Knowing this search for mercy is going on has become one of the clearest expressions of my why. The image of heavily pregnant women wandering the streets asking everyone, everywhere, "Where can I find mercy?" guts me every time. Sometimes it takes a question with a double meaning to bring our purpose into sharp focus.

THE CHOSEN BATTLE

One woman's search for mercy is a window into a much deeper, widespread crisis. Around the world, childbirth is still fraught with danger, and we must not underestimate the scale of what so many families are facing. The reasons behind maternal and newborn deaths are layered and complex, but that does not make them any less urgent to address. In an article my son Ian published after he and his wife Rose moved to the Philippines as newlyweds, he wrote,

> The battle my wife and I have specifically chosen is not against an over-medicalized culture or unnecessary interventions in childbirth care. Instead, it is against a complete lack of childbirth care. It is against death and disease in their worst form: when the medical needs of women and children are met with apathy and neglect.

MIDWIVES AS ONE SOLUTION

If we believe that mothers and babies truly matter, that their lives, safety, and dignity are not negotiable, then we must also ask: Who is best positioned to walk with them during one of life's most vulnerable transitions?

There is a well-documented need for more midwives everywhere in the world, and midwives have been found to be a viable and evidence-based solution to the current maternity care crisis. Based on this evidence, one of my life's purposes is to build and support midwife-led birth centers in low-resource, high-mortality areas, and to train more midwives to save lives worldwide.

And now, midwifery is more relevant than ever. Aligned with best practice guidelines that prioritize protecting the normal physiology of birth, as well as up-to-date technology and skills to respond effectively to birth complications, midwives offer an answer in a time of growing crisis in maternity care. This is not a new answer, but one rooted in generations of wisdom, skill, and presence. Midwifery is not an emerging trend. It's a proven care model that has sustained communities for centuries.

Through Mercy In Action, we've seen firsthand how midwife-led care transforms outcomes. In the Philippines, a low-resource, disaster-prone archipelago in Southeast Asia, our Mercy In Action built and sponsored birth centers have welcomed over 18,000 babies into the world, and counting. Most of our families live with risk factors many would consider insurmountable: malnutrition, poverty, unemployment, limited access to basic emergency healthcare, and frequent housing crises caused by natural disasters.

And yet, for more than three decades, our Mercy In Action birth centers have documented maternal and newborn survival rates that are four times better than the national average for the country of the Philippines. It's not because we have unlimited resources. These results have been achieved in simple, out-of-hospital birth centers run by midwives and funded by donations. The key is that the midwives are well trained, compassionate, and committed to offering respect and evidence-based care to every mother. The outcomes I wrote about in the introduction tell the story.

Elizabeth Gilmore, the late founder of the National College of Midwifery and my mentor and friend, once told me that what was most remarkable about our outcomes was that we achieved them at a particular moment in the history of childbirth when hospital birth with a physician had come to be widely assumed to be the safest option. Elizabeth understood early on what many global health experts are now beginning to acknowledge: Midwives, when supported and empowered, are one of the most effective answers to the crisis in maternity care.

The whole world is starting to notice the efficacy of the midwifery model of care. In 2023, UNESCO placed midwifery on its Representative List of the Intangible Cultural Heritage of Humanity, honoring not only the clinical role of midwives but also their cultural and communal significance. In 2024, the World Health Organization published a groundbreaking report, "Transitioning to Midwifery Models of Care: Global Position Paper." In it, they affirmed that midwife-led continuity models significantly enhance outcomes for women, including satisfaction and safety. The International Confederation of Midwives (ICM)'s theme for its 2026 triennial congress was captured in the title of its global petition, "One Million More Midwives." This growing recognition is a call to invest in midwifery education, to build systems that support midwife-led care, and to prioritize raising a generation of midwives who carry both skill and vision to help solve the maternity care crisis.

WHY MERCY

Mercy is compassion in action, the effort to relieve suffering and the deliberate choice to withhold harm when it is within one's power. This often takes the form of trauma-informed care, recognizing that each person we encounter may carry burdens we cannot see. From the beginning, this mercy work has grown out of a clear understanding that no one should die trying to bring forth life. Even in poverty, even in overlooked places, even when birth is complicated or high-risk, people deserve to be treated with skill, respect, and compassion.

I began my journey into midwifery with a deep sense of purpose. This has anchored me through many professional and personal crises, as well as a few spectacular calamities and setbacks. Yet my why, and our corporate why among my teams, has never wavered since I started in 1980.

Our purpose shapes how we build our birth centers, train midwives, and choose to stay present in communities that others might pass by. Over the years, I've come to believe that mercy is something tangible you can build into everything. It shows up in the decisions we make, the relationships we honor, and the care we provide. And when mercy is paired with excellence, something powerful happens: Lives change, and mothers and babies survive and thrive. Especially on the hardest days, having a purpose that undergirds our actions reminds us what matters most.

THE TEAM APPROACH

Our why shapes how we operate, and, importantly, helps us invite others into this work. We don't want to pressure people to join us out of necessity, but to cast a vision for what is possible so that they join us out of excitement. This work is not just my vision; it's a shared calling among many. As the leader, it is my responsibility to ensure that everyone continues to remember the purpose behind what we do. This is crucial to our team's enjoyment in our work, and it helps in the recruitment and retention of talented staff. Those who are a good fit for our vision understand that everyone is on board for the same reason.

Rules and laws concerning midwifery and midwifery education are constantly shifting. Our world can be rocked by unexpected disasters, pandemics, and political turmoil. Yet, the why of our original mission remains our constant light, guiding our team's navigation. This is especially helpful when, metaphorically speaking, the waters get rough and our ship is pitching on the waves of change and uncertainty.

At this point in my life, I am frequently asked to consult with others who wish to develop maternal child health programs like ours. Whether I am consulted on starting a small nonprofit in Tanzania or applying midwifery theory to practice in a large Swedish university hospital maternity unit, I give the same advice. Clients, patients, staff, and students need to be actively reminded of the purpose behind their business, birth center, or midwifery college. Why was it founded in the first place? What do the leaders and the team players believe about their mission? No matter where we work or serve, we all need to hold each other accountable to the values and guiding principles, whatever they may be, of that fundamental why.

LIVE THE WHY

Each of us comes to birth work along a different path. Some of us followed a sense of calling. Others stepped into this work unexpectedly and found that it captured our hearts. Some enter birth work with timidity and ease in slowly; others jump off the deep end boldly with no looking back. Some midwives come to this calling after their own difficult birth, and others after seeing a sister or friend have an empowering birth. There are some individuals who know they are called to midwifery as a lifelong vocation from a young age, while others begin it as a second career. But no matter how we arrived, what will sustain us is knowing why we do it.

There will be days that are long and heavy. Birth is beautiful, but it can also be demanding and unpredictable. If we don't stay anchored in our purpose, it's easy to become tired, disoriented, or bitter at the sacrifices involved. That's why we must return again and again to the center of our calling. Sacred purpose taps into the whole person of who we are, body, soul, and spirit.

SIMPLE AND COMPLEX

Our why can be both very simple and extremely complex at the same time. The important thing is to take the time to know and understand our personal why. After that, we can figure out how to articulate and personify that why. When we have a firm grasp on it, we will find that we can more easily explain it to others.

Your own why might be deeply spiritual, or more practical. It may be rooted in your own lived experience with pregnancy, birth, and parenting. It might come from a place of justice, empathy, or hope. Whatever it is, name it. Write it down. Speak it aloud. Let it shape your decisions and renew your motivation. Discovering your purpose is a gift you give to yourself that will invariably make your job easier and more fulfilling. Your deeper purpose is unique to you; a person's sense of purpose is as personal as how someone prays.

What I know is that when we keep our why at the center, we can withstand the weight of this work, and learn to carry it with joy. If we live our work as a vocation rather than a job, full of all the devotion and passion we feel in our hearts at our best, we will find that our purpose will sustain us in the worst of times as well.

I live in gratitude and wonderment at the privilege of serving pregnant women and their families as a midwife. Global health experts have documented that roughly one million more midwives are currently needed to meet the needs of mothers and babies around the world. However, simply training more midwives will not solve the problems if those midwives fail to live up to the highest standards of safety and respect, or if they burn out before retirement.

Midwives can be powerful role models as we seek to change the harmful birth culture around us, but only if we are secure in our purpose and dedicated to excellence for the long haul. Starting with a clear focus on why we do what we do helps us see the whole picture and create a strategy from the ground up.

Our why also shapes our behavior in big and small ways. We will examine the character traits that elevate a good midwife into a great midwife in the next chapter.

PAUSE FOR REFLECTION

WHAT IS YOUR PERSONAL REASON FOR BEING INVOLVED IN BIRTH WORK? WHAT FIRST STIRRED YOUR HEART? CAN YOU ARTICULATE YOUR PURPOSE CONCISELY ENOUGH THAT IF SOMEONE ASKED YOU IN AN ELEVATOR WHY YOU DO WHAT YOU DO, YOU COULD TELL THEM BEFORE THE ELEVATOR DOORS OPENED AGAIN?

2
BECOMING THE GIFT WE OFFER

Character cannot be developed in ease and quiet. Only through experiences of trial and suffering can the soul be strengthened, vision cleared, ambition inspired, and success achieved.

— HELEN KELLER

MY PARENTS QUIETLY MODELED PRINCIPLED BEHAVIOR THROUGHOUT their lives. My dad was a highly intelligent man, a rancher who lived by a gentlemanly cowboy code of conduct. He taught me what it meant to live with honor and to look out for your neighbor. For him, it was all about how you treated people; that was the true measure of respect. My mom showed me honesty and warmth in practical ways. She was never happier than when working in customer service roles, where she could brighten someone's day by going the extra mile to make them feel special and cared for. When I reflect on the people my parents were, the way they related to others was an outward sign of something deeper: their character.

Character is one of those elusive qualities that's hard to pin down in words, but unmistakable when you see it. My parents had it. They cultivated an environment around them that naturally encouraged them to be a certain kind of person. Though they were human and therefore imperfect like all of us, both my mother and father radiated an incorruptibility that rose above their modest circumstances and drew others toward their light. Because of who Ray and Mike Allen were and how consistently they lived out their values in their small, rural community, they left an outsized impact on the lives around them.

When my mom died shortly after they had celebrated their sixtieth wedding anniversary, no church in the area could contain the crowd that came to honor her. Her funeral was moved to the local fairgrounds, where more than five hundred people gathered to pay their respects. Three years later, when my father passed, it was the same story. A filled-to-capacity crowd packed into the California State Fairgrounds activity center to remember him.

At both funerals, my siblings and I sat late into the evening listening to story after story, accounts of how our parents' humble character had shaped the lives of those relating the stories. They spoke of defining moments of interaction that affected them, often in deeply transformative ways. One cousin told us how, late one night, he looked at my father's worn cowboy boots by the door and felt a reckoning in his soul. He realized he wanted to walk in those boots, not literally, but in the life of integrity they represented. That moment, gazing at those dusty boots, he said, led him to turn his life around.

THE CHARACTER OF A MIDWIFE

As important as I believe character is, I can't recall ever hearing any experts point to character as part of the solution to improve maternal and newborn health. Yet after many years working as a midwife, I have come to believe character is foundational. It certainly impacts outcomes in small and big ways, and leads me to believe more attention should be paid to our outward expressions of inward character if we want to see positive change in childbirth culture.

Over the years, I've made a study of the character traits that a good midwife must live out, because the behaviors that flow from one's character, whether it be good character, or whether character is lacking, can shape outcomes in profound and lasting ways. A focus on midwives building a strong and ethical character is another secret to good outcomes in birth.

BUILDING CHARACTER

Building character isn't about having all the answers or presenting ourselves as some flawless model of virtue. I write about character not as someone who has mastered it, but as someone still learning and still praying for the grace to live what I say I believe. It is a constant struggle to lay down, day by day, my own less-than-ideal instincts.

No one does this perfectly. We all fall short. Most of us can recall moments when we failed to live up to the character a situation required of us. Those moments can be embarrassing, even mortifying. Perhaps it happens in a meeting, a clinical encounter, or with family around a dinner table. Someone says something that touches a nerve, and before wisdom has time to speak, impatience or anger does. Perhaps it was a moment when you chose pride over humility, or stayed silent when courage was required. The moment passes, but the regret lingers.

Having character means making a daily effort, being constantly committed to growing into the kind of person who can be relied upon when it truly counts. If we embrace the lessons inherent in both the scars of failures and the highs of victory, a stronger character can emerge. The failure itself isn't the final word. What matters is what we do afterward, whether we retreat in shame or lean into the momentary failure to allow it to make us just a bit wiser, a little more honest, and willing to keep learning. Do we apologize and do what we can to make the situation right? Do we determine to work on having better self-control?

It is possible to walk away from character lapses knowing not only what we should have done, but also what we hope to do differently the next time. That steady inward shaping of character is part of the work of midwifery, too.

Character development in any area takes embracing one character trait over and over, and that is humility. Over the years, my awareness of how much I depend on humility to walk this path of service and leadership with integrity has deepened. There is a wonderful story about an entrepreneur who was asked why he was so successful. His response was "Good decisions." The second question was "How do you make good decisions?" His response: "Experience." And then the final question: "How do you get experience?" And his response was: "Bad decisions!" This is how we grow and stay humble at the same time.

WHAT CHARACTER IS (AND ISN'T)

Sometimes people talk about character and attitude like they are the same thing, but they're not, even though both are crucial in birth work. Attitude is our outlook, our mindset, the way we approach people and situations. While we may naturally skew toward a particular attitude type, for most of us on any given day, our attitude is shaped by mood, fluctuating hormones, or even how much sleep we got the night before. Elusive and fleeting, attitude shifts with the weather of our lives.

But character goes deeper. Character is steadier than attitude, more dependable than emotion, and stronger than circadian rhythms. It holds steadfast in the ups and downs of life and does not yield its influence when unexpected curveballs are thrown at us. Our deep inner character shows up when the pressure is on and the stakes are high. It shows up when no one is watching; maybe especially then.

Character is what anchors us when the path gets rough. It's what keeps us speaking up when it's costly or inconvenient, or when the temptation strikes to cover up instead of telling the truth. Character is what helps us remember who we are, who we want to be, and who we are there for.

In his book *Hidden Potential*, Adam Grant puts it this way: "Personality is not your destiny—it's your tendency. Character skills enable you to transcend that tendency to be true to your principles." I find that concept hopeful, because it tells me that even when I fail, I can stay true to my principles. I can tap into my commitment to character and apologize or do whatever else is needed to make the situation right. Just as purpose gives us our why for our lives, character gives us our how to live by.

Because character is not built around a personality type, and it isn't something you either have or you don't, we all have the same opportunity to improve. Character also isn't built overnight. Rather, character is something we construct, brick by brick, over time, as we identify and stay true to our principles based on the things we deem important. It's what we do on hard days, in the choices made in the public eye, and those made in private. It is a decision to be better and do better, both personally and professionally.

The good news is that no matter what good or bad choices we may have made in the past, and regardless of whether our family of origin set a good or bad example of character, we can start building a good character (or renovating a shoddy one) today. Shaping our character is a lifetime commitment, and one worthy of our undertaking. In the big scheme of what we hope to accomplish through our vocation in birth work, our individual character is vitally important.

HOW CHARACTER SHAPES OUTCOMES

My friend Christy, an alumna of our midwifery college, shared this story with me. She had attended a peaceful water birth at home when, just minutes after the birth, she noticed the pool filling with blood. At first, she thought the mother was bleeding, but a quick assessment told her otherwise. The cord had spontaneously snapped right after birth. This is a rare and potentially fatal situation, and the baby was losing blood rapidly. Immediately, Christy clamped the cord and called for emergency services. When the paramedics arrived, she stated clearly for the record that the pale, limp baby had bled out through the cord.

From the back of the ambulance, Christy called ahead to the hospital on her cell phone to tell them to be ready with an immediate blood transfusion. Thanks to her quick actions and the mutually respectful relationship she had forged over the years with the hospital staff, the baby received a blood transfusion immediately upon arrival. The baby survived, without lasting effects. Disaster was averted.

You may think that is a good example of a midwife's skill and foresight, based on good training, and you would be right. But what if her character also may have saved that baby's life?

When she told me the story, I got chills up and down my spine, because I couldn't help recalling a similar story a few years earlier. It was the same complication, except that in this instance the cord clamp was not fastened properly and came loose. The result was the same, though; the baby lost a significant amount of blood from his cut umbilical cord before the situation was discovered. The midwife in charge re-clamped the cord and called for an ambulance when she discovered the problem, but she hid what had happened, perhaps afraid of getting into trouble. This baby died.

According to records later made public in the case, it seemed the midwife had not shared the facts of the case with the ambulance crew or the receiving hospital. Not knowing what caused the baby's pale, limp condition, valuable time was wasted while the doctors were running tests and chasing differential diagnoses. No one at the hospital knew the baby needed an urgent blood transfusion. After the baby died, an autopsy revealed the truth, but it was too late.

The midwives in both of these stories had the same skill set. They both noticed the bleeding, clamped the cord, and called for transport to the hospital. But one midwife told the truth and the other did not. The outcomes were drastically different, and the difference came down to character. One midwife exhibited the character traits of honesty, accountability, and integrity. The other midwife did not.

A baby paid with his life. And the parents and their entire extended family will live with the grief and loss forever.

CAN CHARACTER BE TAUGHT?

A few years back, I became disturbed to realize I was hearing stories more and more often about community midwives who were making choices that raised concerns, such as altering charts, telling students to ignore vital signs, and minimizing mistakes. At the same time, I heard frequent stories about midwives who were making admirable choices in difficult situations, such as self-reporting an error in a drug dosage, correcting course based on emerging evidence, or publicly apologizing for a misunderstanding or wrongdoing within the birth community.

It left me wondering: Can character be taught? Can our midwifery college nurture the kind of formation that not only builds skills but shapes trustworthiness? Can behavior based on inner integrity, expressed through character traits, be cultivated in midwives-in-training?

That curiosity stayed with me until it took root and became something practical, and this is where strategy came in. With my team at the Mercy In Action College of Midwifery, I created a curriculum thread of character traits that now weaves through all four years of our midwifery college. We named this curriculum "The Character of a Midwife," and we tie it directly to birth outcomes.

The concept is simple but profound: to help students recognize how character shows up, for better or worse, in the day-to-day realities of midwifery practice, impacting real choices, real decisions, and real outcomes. We want our students to see behaviors based on character, not as abstract ideals or theory, but as a stark example of theory-to-practice case studies.

Throughout all four years of our college, we hold classes where we ask our midwifery students to reflect on how expressing a particular individual character trait could lead to a better outcome for their clients or patients. As we examine twenty-eight distinct character traits, we also ask the opposite: What happens when a midwife doesn't walk in the character trait we are studying? How does character (or the lack thereof) impact trust, safety, and well-being for those being cared for by that provider?

When we launched the new curriculum, our goal was to link the inner workings of character traits to the outer results, and it didn't take long before students began to see the connection. They quickly realized that doing the hard work of building good character isn't optional. The way character has the power to influence better birth outcomes was apparent from the start; we had opened the door to a new understanding of what makes a midwife safe and respectful.

Soon students began sharing their own stories and examples in class. Their conversations sparked ideas and a desire to bring about real change in healthcare. Through their storytelling, I saw them begin to reflect deeply, ruminating together on the different expressions of character they were seeing in real life. Connecting the dots, they realized that a strong character empowers midwives to give their very best. What would it look like, they postulated, if a system could be built and sustained on mutual trust and respect and all the other positive character traits?

For all of us, these classes have been a steady reminder that good outcomes don't just happen, and they don't hinge solely on what we know (medical and midwifery knowledge) or what we can do (skills and talents). It's more nuanced than that. Outcomes will always depend on many factors, but who we are and how we operate in the world make a big difference.

Because we recognize that character is more likely to be caught than taught, we encourage our students to continually share these stories with each other, considering what they are seeing in their apprenticeship in light of their Character of a Midwife curriculum. A pattern begins to emerge as stories are passed around and decisions, behaviors, and attitudes are analyzed. Character-based choices do have an impact on birth outcomes. Within this framework, the instinct to do the right thing is recognized and praised.

WIDER IMPACT

How we see the world impacts our credibility in a prenatal clinic setting. The decisions we make can change the course of events in a medical emergency. The character traits we bring to the birth room affect not only us, but our relationships with medical and midwifery peers. Ultimately, for better or worse, our character may impact the entire birth community where we practice.

Midwives are often highly regarded and looked up to in their communities. Our actions affect those around us, including the home birth community, birth centers and hospitals, and the individual doctors, nurses, doulas, and other midwives who comprise our community.

When we choose to do the hard work of cultivating our better nature, especially in the hard moments or under pressure, we're doing more than being professional. We're helping to build a culture of safety and solidarity that will send ripples of positive change out into the world.

Both aspiring midwives and seasoned professionals need to take this seriously—we all contribute to the health of our communities, so don't underestimate your influence.

SPECIFIC TRAITS

At our midwifery college, we examine twenty-eight character traits over the four-year program. To delve into all of them here would be to write another book, so let's walk through just a few of these traits together so that you can get the idea. At the end of this chapter, I will list all twenty-eight traits that we focus on so you can study them too.

The Character Traits of Accountability and Honesty

Let's begin our look through a few important character traits by focusing on honesty and its close neighbor, accountability.

I often tell stories about mistakes I have made and how I have handled them. This is because I want our students to know that human beings make mistakes, but we can own those mistakes and correct them. I tell them it is better to build a habit of truth-telling when it's something small than try to find the courage to tell the truth when it's something big.

Accountability is the willingness to take responsibility for our choices. It means doing what we say we will do, and when we make a mistake, not hiding from it, but calling on our humility and courage to name it and make amends.

A midwife who practices accountability becomes someone that others can rely on. Clients feel safe. Peers trust them. And the systems they work within become stronger because of their presence.

Accountability isn't just about following protocols. It's about deep integrity. It's about owning our actions, even when there may be unpleasant consequences. When we take responsibility without making excuses, we open the door to the increased likelihood of good outcomes. In our honesty, we model what it looks like to be both professional and human. And we create space for trust to flourish.

One sign of healthy accountability is welcoming peer review and post-birth reflections, not as a place for defensiveness, but as a chance to grow. Each time we choose accountability, we're choosing to live with integrity, and that's the foundation upon which every character trait is built.

Honesty is a prerequisite to walking in accountability. Accountability is taking responsibility for our actions after the fact. Honesty is what happens in the moment, choosing to speak the truth, especially when it costs us something. One trait acknowledges what's been done; the other refuses to hide it. Both are necessary if we want to change birth culture and improve birth outcomes. There is no substitute for practicing with integrity. So much can be accomplished only when we have earned the right to be trusted.

Honesty is the bedrock of trust. It's about being truthful, sincere, and transparent, not just with others but also with ourselves. Although we will not always get every decision right, honesty keeps us grounded and helps protect the people in our care.

The opposite is also true: Once a person has been caught lying, it is hard to trust them again. A healthcare worker who makes changes to a chart or an insurance form to protect themselves, hide an error, or make an illegal profit is committing fraud. Once you have been caught fabricating details on any official form, anything you record in the future will be open to suspicion. Trust must be sacred in our line of work.

I say all of this while acknowledging that the temptation to protect oneself is real. When we make a mistake or act outside of our protocols or scope of practice, that can easily lead to small fibs or lying by omission in charting or when referring a case. However, even small lies and omissions can be harmful. Resisting the temptation to lie or cover up a mistake is one sign of a strong character. If we always tell the truth even in small ways, people are more likely to believe us when something really consequential comes along. Honesty invites trust, and trust lays the foundation for safe and respectful birth. As midwives, we have many character tests; being honest and accountable are tests we must pass every time. When honesty builds the bridge of trust, compassion and mercy can cross it to offer care that is safe and helps bring about the outcomes we hope to see.

The Character Traits of Compassion and Mercy

Compassion is what happens when we allow ourselves to be moved by another person's suffering. It's more than feeling sorry or feeling pity. Compassion is about feeling another's pain and staying present, letting love move us to action on their behalf.

In birth work, we witness people in their most vulnerable moments. Years ago, I helped a young mother who had no one by her side. Libby was essentially alone in the world; she even drove herself to the birth center when contractions became regular. Her labor was long, her back ached, and fear clung to her like sweat. Seeing that she had no one with her, I stayed right by her side all night, offering water through a straw, doing hip squeezes for hours, and wringing out cold washcloths for her forehead. A midwife's loving presence through a long, dark night of pain can do more than any epidural, with no harmful side effects. After the birth, she leaned in and whispered to me, "Never in my life have I felt surrounded by love—until now, here."

Another time, I received a gut-wrenching call to come immediately to check on one of my pregnant clients. Birgitta had just been given the news that her young husband was dead, killed in a plane crash. I chose to walk beside her in her worst nightmare, and in spite of a busy schedule and a family of my own, I made a point to check on her every day for months throughout the rest of that long, lonely pregnancy. Through the grief-filled hours of Birgitta's labor pains and the weeks of postpartum recovery with her little fatherless baby girl, I stayed close and available. I will never forget that time, being willing to take some of her suffering onto myself, though I could hardly bear it. I often wonder how much pain a human heart can endure. There is nothing more essential at times like these than love and tenderness, practiced in the present moment for someone in desperate need.

Compassion is not weakness. It's one of our strongest tools. It softens the edges of suffering, reminding people that they are not forgotten. In our line of work, compassion can make a difficult birth bearable and an impossible situation surmountable.

Mercy, a word often used interchangeably with compassion, is actually defined as compassion extended to someone whom it is in your power to harm. We may not realize the enormous power we hold as healthcare workers, and that power can either heal or harm. The way we speak, the way we touch, the way we respond to people who are hurting or scared—all of this can either reinforce human dignity or cause deep and lasting wounds. This is especially true for people living on the margins of society, who may arrive into care dreading the power imbalance. Obstetric violence has been identified as one of the many ways that a woman may have her human rights violated during labor and delivery, and it often happens due to a lack of mercy on the part of the providers.

Mercy isn't just a part of what my team values, it's our very mission. It is intentionally in our name; it is in the DNA of our organization. Our Mercy In Action staff, on both sides of the world, feel that mercy is the beating heart of all we are called to do. Mercy turns medical care into a healing presence, and helps restore a sense of worth to those who have long been overlooked and denied. We hope that our mercy-infused actions remind those we serve of the *imago Dei* inside of them.

Years ago, in my early days of working in the Philippines, I volunteered at a provincial hospital where poor people were often treated quite harshly. One day, a woman named Floribeth arrived in labor to give birth to her eighth baby, but it was discovered that the baby was dead inside of her. The fetal demise had caused her to become ill, and the diagnosis was sepsis.

Sepsis is a serious form of infection and is one of the top four reasons that women worldwide die around the time of childbirth. Once called childbed fever, sepsis was much feared before the advent of antibiotics in the 1940s. It was the reason my own grandmother was orphaned just days after her birth in 1896 in America.

I was shocked when a doctor came in and began to berate Floribeth for having so many children, saying she was so poor that she had no business getting pregnant. To my horror, he told her angrily that it would be her own fault if she died. After the doctor left, I went over to Floribeth and offered her a cup of water, gently lifting her shoulders to help her take a sip. As long as I live, I will never forget the look on her face. To me, it was just a small kindness: a drink of water! But her response utterly broke my heart. It was as if I had done something wonderful and unbelievable. Her gratitude was so raw, so totally out of proportion to the deed. The look in her eyes shattered me. I realized in that moment Floribeth may have spent a lifetime deprived of human kindness.

The next day when I arrived at the hospital I immediately went to check on Floribeth, and I received a rude awakening to the ways things worked in poor rural hospitals in the Philippines at that time. Though her condition was worsening and she was now desperately ill, they had not yet started her on antibiotics because no one in her family could afford to buy them. I went immediately to fill her prescription, and in the days ahead, I came often to pray for her. Tucked into the corner on a dirty cot, Floribeth's fever left her drifting in and out of consciousness, and I knew she might not survive. When she did eventually begin to recover, she told me she had heard my prayers, even in the times she could not respond, and believed she had been healed by the mercy she felt coming from me into her very being while I prayed.

Mercy has the power to reach past the situation and into the pain. It doesn't ask if someone deserves it. Sometimes what brings forth healing isn't just medicine. It's mercy that makes someone feel valued when the world has devalued them. Maybe it is their first taste of love. In my experience, mercy is often viewed as counterculture in places where only those who are compliant, without addictions or quirks, and can pay in full, are afforded respectful maternity care.

Mercy also shows that we acknowledge everyone falls short and that people are more than their worst moments. It takes grit to show gentleness when you're exhausted and a client or one of their family members is abusive toward you. It takes strength to extend mercy, especially when forgiveness needs to be involved.

Sometimes I am asked, "Aren't you afraid people will take advantage of you?" My answer is: "How can someone take advantage of what I am giving away freely?"

Compassion and mercy should not be reserved only for the clients we serve; we need to extend this deliberate tenderness to everyone on our team. Students need it in large doses when they are first starting out. Mercy and compassion shape the behavior of future midwives and may be what helps them stay in the work long-term.

We can also show compassion to the receiving hospital workers during a home-to-hospital transfer. The hospital-based providers may not understand your system of care, and the uncertainty of the unfamiliar situation may feel scary for them, too. Empathy is a sister to compassion, and it is often helpful to try to see things through someone else's perspective, especially when it is vastly different from your own. This is a sign of mature character.

To keep showing up year after year, decade after decade, with one's compassion and mercy still intact requires more than good intentions and passion; it takes resilience and perseverance, the strength to stay the course.

The Character Traits of Resilience and Perseverance

The summer I met Scott, he was homesteading in Alaska. I was visiting mutual friends, and we fell in love. I did not leave for business college until early October, and consequently, he left town late in the season, loading his Grumman cargo canoe with winter supplies and heading down the Chatanika River toward his remote cabin. Three days into the trip, winter caught him. The river froze and held his canoe fast. He hiked the rest of the way to the cabin, several miles as the crow flies, then returned with an axe the next day, only to find the river had overflowed and frozen again, sealing the canoe under two feet of ice. All winter long, he made the long trek in subzero weather to chop it out by hand. He knew that if he did not free it before spring breakup, the river would take it. Perseverance, as I have come to understand it, often looks like this: quiet, hard work, sometimes with real risk, done day after day, choosing not to give up until the thing that matters is finally brought through. That canoe is still in use today, used by our son and grandchildren in Fairbanks. It bears the scars of axe marks along both edges, a testament to a "never say die" spirit.

I gave a lecture recently to a class of seminary doctoral students from several countries. All of them worked under difficult conditions, some worse than mine, as their countries were at war, but they were all significantly younger than I was. During the question-and-answer session, they expressed admiration for my long years in ministry. One of the students raised his hand and asked me, "Don't you ever want to give up?"

People think that because I have done what I have done for so long, I must be immune to hopelessness. Actually, I fight against it all the time. "Yes," I answered truthfully, "I wanted to give up only yesterday!" I then related a story about a particularly difficult morning the day before, and the moment I thought to myself, "I don't have to keep doing this. I could do something easier. Why do I put myself through this?" But then I immediately reminded myself I had not signed up for easy. I had signed up for loving people and saving lives. "Oh, right! Back to work," I said to myself.

It happens—we all have days we want to give up, to stop chopping at the ice. Anyone involved in birth work (or any intense ministry or profession, for that matter) is bound to have such moments. The important thing to remember is that wanting to quit and actually quitting are two different things.

Resilience and perseverance work together to sustain meaningful change. Resilience allows us to recover when hardship knocks the wind out of us. Perseverance is the steady choice to continue, even when the path is long and uphill. And then there is a close cousin to both, tenacity, which is the resolve to hold fast when resistance presses in and letting go feels tempting. If we hope to lead change and shape outcomes over the long haul, we will need all these character traits in generous measure. Perseverance carries us forward year after year, resilience helps us recover when we stumble, and tenacity ensures we do not loosen our grip along the way.

Many experts have explored what gives a person the strength to persevere and respond to difficulties with resilience and tenacity. Psychologist Angela Duckworth describes this essential quality with one simple word: grit.

Grit is defined as the unwavering courage and resolve to keep going, no matter how rough the way. Grit is about rising after setbacks, staying focused on long-term goals, and pushing through obstacles with steady determination. Grit weaves together passion with perseverance, and many times is what helps us finish the race we start, no matter how hard the climb or how long the distance.

Grit explains why some people are able to rise again after unimaginable grief, recalibrate after earth-shattering failure, and keep choosing hope when things feel hopeless. This is essential for midwives, who face innumerable sleepless nights, complications and emergencies they didn't see coming, as well as losses that can't always be prevented. It is the strength of spirit to recover from any adversity. When experiencing disappointment, loss, or tragedy, it gives us the impetus to keep looking until we find the hope and courage to carry on.

One midwife student I trained, Lynnel, experienced a traumatic birth early in her apprenticeship. It shook her to her core. For weeks afterward, she questioned whether she was cut out for this calling. But instead of walking away, she pressed in. She sought counsel, processed the experience, and cried with her mentors. She returned to study birth complications again and again because she wanted to understand what had happened and what could possibly happen. And then, Lynnel stepped back into the birth room.

Her next client was a young mother who carried a lot of fear about birth. Lynnel cared for her with such tenderness, steadiness, and grace that by the end of the birth, when mother and baby were resting quietly, I told Lynnel, "You have what it takes." She never looked back and practiced midwifery with joy (and grit) for another thirty-five years until her death.

Many of us overcome obstacles by tapping into a deep well of faith that helps us endure. Others turn to trusted friends and family for comfort and to be reminded of our self-identified purpose. I find that humor helps a great deal, especially the kind that lets me laugh at myself. I try to take life seriously without taking myself too seriously. Small moments of levity often serve as a buffer against the weight of sorrow and ward off despair. Alongside prayer, a sense of humor is probably one of my greatest tools for staying resilient and mentally healthy.

Resilience and perseverance are essential in midwifery and birth work. When we allow hard experiences to deepen our character instead of defeating us, we become the kind of presence others can count on. Hard things can leave us scarred, but scars are not to be feared. Those hard things can also ground us and help us mature in ways nothing else can.

However, and I must say, there are appropriate times not to persevere as well. I have had to give up some ideas that did not work out and end programs that have failed to produce results. Regrouping and reassessing a given situation is not the same as quitting. At times, with proper consideration and consultation, we may realize it is time to fold a program or walk away from a toxic interpersonal situation. There are times we may be forced to let go of some part of our venture, as there are circumstances exerting pressure beyond our control. At times, I have chosen to step back or turn things over when a leader under me sought to assert control over one of our clinical sites, believing that engaging in conflict on the mission field is contrary to the heart of the mission. What is important is that we never relinquish our tenacious hold on the main purpose of our lives, our why for doing the work. How many times has the thought crossed my mind to give up? Too many to count. When have I quit the big-picture vision of this work? Exactly never.

Over the years, even through failures and the heartbreaking losses of birth centers that we started to fire, floods, conflict, and corruption, the work has endured. The big vision, of showing love in practical ways by helping mothers and babies survive and thrive, and training midwives to do the same, has remained steady throughout my adult life. I often credit any success I've had to a certain Allen family determination and the famous Penwell never-say-die attitude. But if I am honest, I would have to say that what has allowed me to keep showing up, underneath the perseverance, resilience, tenacity, and grit, has been the character trait of courage. I get lots of chances to practice it.

The Character Trait of Courage

In 2006, I was living on an island in the Philippines, where the only way off was a ninety-minute ferry ride across a strait of the ocean. A typhoon had just passed through, and the sea was rough as our small *bangka* boat left the harbor. When the boat reached the open ocean, it began hitting big waves hard, again and again, until it started to break apart. Above the roar of the diesel engine and the crashing of waves, I heard a loud BOOM as the bamboo outrigger broke off and punctured through the side of the boat.

As the ferry rapidly took on water and sank, panic stripped away all restraint from the passengers. Screaming people fought for life vests, pushing, shoving, and climbing over one another. Courage to me in that moment meant holding onto my values; saving myself would have required becoming someone I was not, because long ago I had decided that I would never save my life at the expense of someone else losing their life. So with no certainty of survival, I chose not to fight for a life vest. As people stepped on me in mass panic, I protected my head and proceeded to try to get a message to Scott on my cell phone, though the signal out at sea was not strong enough for a call to go through. In the end, I just had time to send my husband a text message—"Sinking. I love you"—before we were underwater. Having no life vest, I fully expected that to be the day I died. And though I had experienced a momentary panic when the boat first started breaking apart, now that I had decided death was a certainty, I experienced a wonderful calm and felt strangely at peace.

Like most of us, I don't relish the times I need courage, but this character trait has marked my life continuously over the years through experiences I have encountered, endured, and survived. There were times I needed courage for things that only felt scary, but at other times, I drew upon courage for situations that were truly dangerous and demanded every ounce I could muster.

Unlike the ferry sinking, which was immediate and dramatic, I had lots of time to process the fear that gripped me as I prepared to lead a team of midwives into the massive destruction caused by a super typhoon in 2013. This was a humanitarian disaster on a massive scale, and as the leader of Mercy In Action, I had made the decision that we would be first responders. Our role was to set up birth tents at ground zero, because all the health facilities where babies could be born in the area had been demolished by the almost two hundred mile-per-hour winds and subsequent storm surge that had destroyed everything in its path.

In this situation, there were plenty of legitimate reasons to feel afraid. Death was everywhere. Over six thousand people had perished in the storm, and in the days that followed, thousands more were at risk of dying from their injuries, thirst, and slow starvation. Infrastructure was destroyed on two islands. Hospitals were flattened, military bases destroyed, and entire communities left without shelter, food, or potable water. Even the prison walls had collapsed, releasing inmates into a landscape already steeped in chaos, fear, and desperation.

We would be camping in tents, with no doors to lock and no electricity for lights. I was deeply apprehensive. I had some idea of what I would witness, and though willing, I knew I would see things I could never unsee. Having responded to small disasters before, I was experienced and prepared, yet this disaster was larger, darker, and more devastating than anything any of us on my team had ever experienced.

It was courage that helped me board the plane in Manila, land on a broken airstrip on Leyte Island, drive down into an apocalyptic scene, and pitch a group of tents where mothers would soon give birth. Courage showed up in the way our quickly assembled team worked so well together, holding space for life to begin in a place saturated with death.

Right before I left, I had called my daughter-in-law Manga to confess my fear. As we ended the call, she said to me, "Put on your game face, Vic." It was good advice for a leader, because fear can be contagious, so we must be discerning about who we let see it. But as we rendezvoused with our ambulance driver at the broken airport and drove deep into the scenes of utter destruction along the path of the killer typhoon, I took a reading on my heart and was surprised to find it calm, and my mind still fairly sound. The fear was gone.

We arrived in the coastal community of Dulag, where we had a contact, around sunset, and the mayor came out and invited us to stay, as they had no medical assistance yet of any kind. (We later found out Dulag was where the eye of the storm made landfall.) At twilight, we set up our tents and began caring for hurting people. I was so busy and focused, I did not have time to feel afraid. As the sun set on a land that would not get electricity restored for months, I found that compassion had replaced fear, and in spite of the darkness, deprivation, and heartache surrounding us, I felt settled. Mercy and compassion had proven to be stronger than fear.

Courage is the quiet strength that helps us do the right thing, even and maybe especially when we are afraid. In midwifery, courage doesn't always look like dramatic heroism. Sometimes we are called on to save lives, and that takes courage, certainly, but more often, courage looks like speaking up when something doesn't feel right, or admitting when we don't know what to do next.

Courage also shows up in how we handle mistakes. I've seen a midwife tremble as she began to speak during a peer review, confessing an error she'd made. Her voice shook, her eyes brimmed with tears, but she told the truth. Afterward, someone hugged her and said, "Good job owning your stuff with humility and guts."

Courage is not about the absence of fear; rather, it's about acting even in the presence of it. It's about choosing integrity, even when there's risk involved. And it's what allows every other virtue to rise when tested. Consider the wisdom of C. S. Lewis, who said, "Courage is not simply one of the virtues, but the form of every virtue at the testing point." Lewis reminds us that true courage is what gives voice to all other virtues when we face our most difficult moments.

In this work, we often find ourselves right there, at the testing point. May we choose courage, again and again, to embody the character traits that matter most to achieving the good outcomes we want to see.

Oh, and mine was the only distress signal sent that day from the sinking ferry, and Scott received my message—to his great consternation. He ran to alert the boatmen at the dock, who did not know about the maritime disaster, but at Scott's insistence, finally believed him and alerted the Coast Guard. A rescue boat was eventually dispatched to find us. By grace, no lives were lost at sea that day.

A PERSONAL INVENTORY

When we discuss the character needed to be a great midwife, we are never just talking in abstractions or theory. Within Mercy In Action, we encourage our midwives and students alike to take regular personal inventory and reflect on the kind of person they want to be, rather than focusing solely on building a skill set. We prioritize developing the kind of inner steadiness, integrity, and fortitude that I believe great midwifery demands.

Character always matters. It shapes how families remember their birth story, and whether they feel respected, valued, and empowered at the end of their childbearing year. It colors our professional relationships with other providers and either eases or hinders our ability to collaborate and refer for specialty care when needed. Our behavior, based on our character, influences how our own families feel about the sacrifices we ask them to make along with us in order to live out this calling. The way we show up, especially when we're tired, overwhelmed, unsure, or frightened, shapes the entire culture around us.

Each of us will find that our character needs to be custom-built, and we are the builders. It will be shaped by individual circumstances, honed by hard knocks and polished by sheer will and determination. A universal truth is that the most growth occurs in the most challenging places, and character is revealed most when doing the right thing comes at a cost.

Do you long to change the world in a way that meets a felt need for millions of women having babies all over the world? The things that threaten to lead our good intentions astray are often short-term discomforts and annoyances, but the qualities we call character endure over the long term, such as courage, honesty, mercy, and resilience. These characteristics, along with a humble sense of purpose and vocation, can lead us to the places we value most in ourselves and provide us with the tools we need to serve others well. People of character tend to be humble and rarely call attention to themselves, yet they leave a lasting legacy in the lives they touch.

LOVE AND CHARACTER

We don't hesitate to talk about love within the culture Mercy In Action has built. Love, though not usually considered a character trait, is foundational, shaping a person's thoughts, behaviors, and actions. Love finds expression through character. While the word is rarely spoken in medical circles, we recognize the importance of forming and maintaining close, caring relationships with those we serve, and those we serve beside.

While opportunities to build character will arise unbidden throughout our lifetime, we can make a conscious effort today to develop a strategy for paying attention to our character and intentionally forming habits that will keep us on track to continue walking in our deepest purpose. In my teaching and mentoring, I try to convey my own hard-earned lessons that love is a necessary foundation for anything good we want to accomplish. We can and should start by committing to improving our ability to love people, and that will help us add the other character traits to the equation.

So while love for our clients and patients is essential in midwifery, love alone is not enough. In *Somewhere Safe with Somebody Good*, Jan Karon reflects that even where love is present, character is still required:

“You love him, I can see it.”

“More than anything.”

That alone should be enough, he thought, but of course it never is. Courage has to come in there somewhere, and perseverance and forbearance and patience, and all the rest. A job of work, as Uncle Billy would say, but worth it and then some.

PAUSE FOR REFLECTION

CAN YOU RECALL A TIME WHEN A MIDWIFE OR OTHER BIRTH ATTENDANT'S CHARACTER TRAITS, EITHER POSITIVE OR NEGATIVE, DIRECTLY IMPACTED THE OUTCOME OF A BIRTH? WHAT WAS THE RESULT? FROM THE LIST BELOW, PICK ONE OR TWO CHARACTER TRAITS YOU WANT TO START WORKING ON STRENGTHENING TODAY. THEN COME BACK TO THIS LIST AGAIN AND AGAIN; KEEP DOING SO UNTIL YOU HAVE FOCUSED ON THEM ALL.

THE CHARACTER OF A MIDWIFE

1. Accountability
2. Compassion
3. Confidence
4. Cooperation
5. Courage
6. Curiosity
7. Empathy
8. Encouragement
9. Excellence
10. Flexibility
11. Generosity
12. Grace
13. Gratitude
14. Honesty
15. Hospitality
16. Humility
17. Integrity
18. Justice
19. Kindness
20. Leadership
21. Mercy
22. Perseverance
23. Purposefulness
24. Resilience
25. Respect
26. Self-discipline
27. Service
28. Thoughtfulness

The 28 Character Traits Specifically Examined in Mercy In Action College of Midwifery

3
ABUNDANT HOSPITALITY

Service is black and white. Hospitality is color.

— WILL GUIDARA

AT 30,000 FEET OVER THE PACIFIC OCEAN, I HELPED A WOMAN DELIVER her baby. As the only qualified person on board a Korean Air flight from San Francisco to Seoul, I had about thirty minutes to assess the available medical supplies and to create some measure of privacy before the baby came. Seo-yoon was traveling alone and was understandably frightened when sudden, precipitous labor began halfway into a twelve-hour transpacific flight. I realized right away one of my roles would be to dial down the panic and denial of the flight attendants and of the mother herself and keep everyone calm, even as my mind raced to identify ways to "MacGyver" the situation.

After the baby was born safely, I made sure Seo-yoon was given food and a warm drink while she nursed her baby. During the remaining four hours before landing, I sat beside her, monitoring vital signs, and we talked. She told me that in her two previous deliveries, she had been treated rudely and separated from her baby for hours after birth. Despite her initial embarrassment, she realized this was her best birth ever! Beaming, she said she had never been treated so well or given such loving, kind care. What could easily have been a traumatic experience became something very different.

There is remarkable power in giving people more than they expect. Hospitality, at its heart, is about crafting an experience. A person's experience, though intangible, is still deeply felt. But I believe it's more than just a feeling, and we don't have to leave it to chance. Hospitality can be taught, measured, and woven into a purposeful plan of care. In fact, I am convinced it is one of the often-overlooked forces behind the consistently excellent birth outcomes we see in our Mercy In Action birth centers.

In the previous chapters, we've explored how birth outcomes are shaped by a strong sense of purpose and the character we bring to the work. Now, I want to share another secret I've discovered. Mothers' and babies' health and survival are also profoundly influenced by our willingness to offer truly unusual and unexpected hospitality. As you read, think of how each way of providing hospitality may influence outcomes in your own settings.

HOLISTIC APPROACH

The metrics of physical outcomes in childbirth are routinely tracked, yet they tell only part of the story. Emotional well-being plays a critical role in physical health and recovery. Recognizing this connection is central to a truly holistic approach. Holistic healthcare is a comprehensive understanding of well-being that considers the interconnectedness of a person's physical, mental, emotional, social, and spiritual aspects.

When we incorporate an element of hospitality that impacts all these systems, we have the opportunity to offer something far more meaningful than what is run-of-the-mill in pregnancy care. This kind of approach tends to touch something deep in both giver and receiver, bringing joy to this sacred work and elevating the experience while also improving the physical outcomes.

Healthcare that attends to the whole person has the power to leave lasting impressions that build trust and foster inner strength and healing. Being treated with kindness truly matters. How we make someone feel can directly influence their well-being throughout pregnancy, birth, postpartum healing, and the early years of parenting.

Most midwives and doulas know that a mother who feels safe is more likely to labor effectively. A family that feels welcomed into a clinic space is more likely to return for care, follow advice, and trust their provider when it matters most. A warm and gracious attitude on the part of their midwife or doctor can make it easier to call that provider in the middle of the night to voice a concern. The simple act of offering hospitality can relax tension and reduce the fight-or-flight response in someone who has been previously traumatized, and these emotional aspects can play an outsized role in achieving a good outcome in birth.

OPENHEARTED PROTOCOLS

Hospitality may not be listed in your clinical protocols, but it belongs in every midwife's toolkit. Hospitality isn't fluff. It's a foundational quality of openheartedness and welcome that every recipient of maternity care deserves, not just families who can afford boutique care.

For those of us who long to give people the very best during some of the most vulnerable moments of their lives, hospitality is essential to our understanding of high-quality midwifery. Over the years, Mercy In Action has built hospitality into our birth culture, and we have found that this is extremely effective in our goal of empowering women, strengthening families, and reducing maternal and infant morbidity and mortality. This has worked for us everywhere we have built birth centers and clinics, from Alaska to Mexico, from the Philippine Islands to New Mexico and Idaho. It is effective in high-income, high-resource countries and in low-resource countries where maternal and infant mortality rates are high.

Hospitality can be many things; it is multifaceted and endlessly adaptable. It is caring for others with respect and acceptance, making them feel welcome and safe. It is thinking of personalized ways to help the people around you feel that they belong. Hospitality means giving of yourself and your energy selflessly, as an intentional act of service and love. It may also, at times, mean giving of your possessions or forgoing higher earnings, with the hope of offering something meaningful to those who receive your generosity. With hospitality, you lay the foundation for connection, and with the openness and trust that engenders, good birth outcomes are more likely.

THE TIME WE WASTE

I like to think of serving in terms of lavish hospitality. This means embracing not just service but exceptional service that values time spent helping others. While hospitality is often overlooked in health-care settings or viewed as a luxury rather than a necessity, I believe it is a little-known strategy for bringing about positive change in birth culture, which can have a healthy and even lifesaving impact during the childbearing year.

I first gained inspiration for my philosophy of care as a teenager from one of my favorite passages in literature, in the book *The Little Prince*. A fox is explaining to the little prince that it is the time he has "wasted" on his rose that makes this particular rose of incomparable worth to him. The fox explains, "To me, you are still nothing more than a little boy who is just like a hundred thousand other little boys. And I have no need of you. And you, on your part, have no need of me. To you, I am nothing more than a fox like a hundred thousand other foxes. But if you tame me, then we shall need each other. To me, you will be unique in all the world."

The point of this small story is clear: What makes someone special is the care and attention we pour into them. Love, real connection, and real meaning are built through time. Time spent getting to know one another and serving one another. Time spent asking questions and listening deeply to the answer. Within Mercy In Action's culture, we make it a habit to "waste" time on people. It costs nothing but time, yet it makes people feel deeply valued. Of all the ways a person could waste time, spending time accompanying a woman and her family throughout their childbearing journey with extra care and attention is deeply significant.

Optimization is the practice of streamlining systems for maximum efficiency, but in healthcare, it can sometimes come at the cost of human connection. When everything is measured in time saved and schedules met, we risk designing environments that feel cold rather than caring. If you find yourself becoming controlled by the drive for optimization, perhaps it's time to ask yourself if your clients or patients feel like VIPs in the spaces created for them. Because when people feel truly seen and valued, outcomes tend to improve in ways no efficiency model could anticipate. I believe this is proof that love still matters in clinical care.

KING'S TABLE

In the mid-1990s, my husband and I took the lead in helping our church set up a ministry to feed homeless people in the border town of El Paso, Texas. King's Table was a weekly outreach that we set up to turn the way that charity was delivered upside down. Instead of a food line or potluck-style serving, we filled a room with round tables covered in lovely tablecloths to create a café vibe, and we served each guest as if they were in a fine-dining restaurant. One server would deliver individual drinks to a table, greeting each diner, and another would bring the rolls, serving each person from the bread basket as they circled the tables. Another would serve the main dish. Still another would stop by after the meal with dessert. Between courses, the servers were encouraged to sit down at the tables and engage in conversation with the guests.

We could have served everyone more quickly with trays or by lining them up, but speed wasn't the point. Before each meal, we gathered our volunteers to remind them of our true goal: to create as many meaningful personal connections as possible with each guest. We aimed for at least six different team members to interact with and serve each person in some small way. We referred to these moments as touchpoints, each one an opportunity to affirm dignity through a simple, human connection. We wanted each person who attended this King's Table meal to walk away feeling valued, honored, and loved. We were trying to represent well the hands and feet of Christ.

Since many of the people who came were unhoused and living on the streets, they rarely experienced people going out of their way to spend time with them. Even fewer had the chance to linger over a hot meal, served with such meticulous attention to detail. Our deliberate inefficiency was the very strategy that made it powerful as an expression of love and welcome.

Invariably, this deliberate inefficiency would drive some volunteers crazy. Often, a new volunteer who had missed the pre-meal team gathering (where we shared the why behind our methods) would approach me with their ideas to improve our efficiency. I became accustomed to being told that we shouldn't waste so much time and that we should instead line everyone up to spoon food onto their plates as they walked down a row of servers. I would always respond gently by saying, "Yes, your ideas would be more efficient, I agree. But efficiency isn't our goal, and we are not just serving food, we're here to serve love."

This gives you a background and a reference point for how our teams around the world offer birth care. In the same King's Table spirit, our midwives are encouraged to take time with every person who walks through our doors, creating touchpoints of genuine connection and kindness. We want our clinic to feel less like a medical office and more like walking into the home of a friend, where people are known by name, cared for with tenderness, and never rushed. Just as we can set a literal table and serve each guest with dignity, we use that hospitality model in our midwifery.

Imagine my surprise and delight when I was talking to Jennie Joseph of Commonsense Childbirth in the early days of our friendship, and discovered that she uses basically the same strategy in her Florida clinics! Her similar concept is for staff and volunteers to make individual points of contact with each client, as part of The JJ Way of maternity care she developed. At each prenatal appointment, a client is intentionally introduced to several different members of Jennie's team throughout their visit. This may include the receptionist, a doula, a nutritionist, or a volunteer, even before they meet the midwives.

As she described her model to me, Jennie expressed her hope that the client will bond not only with her baby but with her maternity care providers. If each woman forges a connection with at least one of the several clinic team members, that bond, even if it is not with the primary midwife, becomes protective. It builds trust and changes outcomes. Jennie's style of care has been shown in data analysis to eliminate health disparities in preterm-birth outcomes and reduce the number of low-birth-weight babies in at-risk populations.

I remember smiling to myself as Jennie was sharing her model and her outcomes, thinking that this was the King's Table model—blessed inefficiency at its best!

As discussed earlier, the statistical evidence presented in the Introduction reflects decades of lives saved through our midwife-led birth centers in the Philippines, with survival rates roughly four times higher than the national average. At the heart of these outcomes is a sustained practice of hospitality, embodied in the King's Table strategy, which orders relationships in ways that foster trust, dignity, and thriving.

Commonsense Childbirth illustrates this connection by sharing visual data on their website showing prematurity rates that consistently fall below state averages in Florida, with especially notable differences when the data are viewed by race. Outcomes improve most for those who are most in need of care that feels trustworthy and attentive. Taken together with parallel results Mercy In Action is getting, these outcomes suggest that something beyond clinical protocol is at work. I have come to believe there is a particular power in the deliberately inefficient, radically hospitable model that both Jennie's team and my team have implemented, and that this approach may be one of the keys to achieving our desired outcomes in childbirth. The remarkable thing is, it works in both rich and poor countries.

Watch for those touchpoints in your world of birth care, wherever it may be. Build your own King's Table model, and see what happens. You may find, as Jennie and I have, that instructing your team to "waste" time in strategic ways can serve to make your clients and patients feel more special and loved, which in turn can improve their chances of having a positive birth outcome.

OPEN ACCESS

Hospitality lays the foundation for connection, but there is more needed. We remove monetary barriers to starting prenatal care, and this reduces risk factors. Globally, barriers to maternity care extend far beyond money and include distance and transportation, understaffed or overburdened facilities, lack of respectful or culturally safe care, fear of mistreatment, language barriers, legal or documentation status barriers, and the long shadow trauma caused by past harm within health systems. All of these are barriers we are actively working to eliminate.

In my early days as a midwife in Alaska, I dubbed this style of care *open access*, and that is what we call it to this day in the Philippines. Jennie calls it *easy access* in her clinics. Both terms basically mean that we will figure out later how the service will be paid for, and where it is safe to deliver, but we will never deny care in the moment. I like how Jennie explains it: "Pregnancy is the ticket in the door, nothing else. Once you get in and see a midwife, we will help you get everything else sorted."

In our Philippines clinics, which are open twenty-four hours a day with a midwife always on-site, *open access* looks like ushering someone in who knocks on the door at any hour. Sometimes it is a woman in labor who we have never met before. Other times it is someone inquiring about starting prenatal care, and no matter the time, we never tell her to come back during regular office hours, but give her a checkup right then. In a different context, the first contact may be a phone call, in which case we would arrange a prenatal exam for her as soon as possible.

At that first visit, after taking a history and doing an examination, we often help the person to enroll in any available assistance programs or refer her to an obstetrician if it is a high-risk pregnancy. Our top priority is to ensure that anyone who is pregnant receives high-quality care as early as possible, from a provider most appropriate to provide that care, while offering support navigating complex systems that can otherwise be difficult to manage.

The time we "waste" on each person is what makes them precious to us, and it is also, amazingly, often enough to shift outcomes. We see results like less prematurity and healthier babies at birth. Who knew that intentional inefficiency is a strategy that works so well! This may seem mind-bending to those who prize efficiency above all else, but the midwife who understands hospitality knows that time spent in deliberate unhurriedness like this is time well spent.

The spirit of hospitality leads us to be discerning and never to miss the big picture. This requires a regular review of our purpose and clarity on our goals. And sometimes, it begins with something as simple as a bowl of soup.

SHARING SOUP

I remember a young woman who arrived late for her first appointment at our birth center in Alaska. Yvonne had driven 95 miles with a malfunctioning car heater to get to her appointment and arrived cold, discouraged, and with frost in her hair, having scraped ice condensation off the inside of the windshield the whole way. With worried eyes, she told me that she did not have money for a pregnancy test and had already been denied an appointment to start prenatal care at another clinic because she lacked health insurance.

We could have told her we were closed at that moment for the lunch hour, or started by handing her a clipboard with a stack of intake forms to fill out. But instead, we ladled soup into a bowl and handed it to her with a spoon and an invitation to sit with us and eat. It wasn't anything fancy, but it was a real and heartfelt invitation into fellowship. In that moment, Yvonne's shoulders relaxed and her eyes filled with tears. The intended message came through loud and clear to Yvonne: You are safe here. We will not turn you away. There will be time later to fill out intake forms, confirm your pregnancy, and everything else needed to initiate care.

Sharing food in unexpected places and unforeseen ways can go a long way toward making a person feel welcome and at home in your presence. Hospitality sees the whole person, rather than just the pregnant belly, and asks what they need to truly thrive.

Abundant hospitality means we throw open our hearts without measuring love in specific amounts. It's a way of serving that chooses to see each person as worthy of a little extra time, a little more kindness, and a welcome that has no edge or limit. It's care in the spirit of the good Samaritan, who, after rescuing a wounded man, told the innkeeper, "Take care of him, and whatever more you spend, I will repay you." This is the kind of hospitality that has the power to change outcomes because it puts no limits on the cost.

IDENTIFYING NEED

If you are working among women living in poverty, hospitality shown through the sharing of food should be a meaningful part of prenatal care, because nothing complicates a pregnancy quite like not having enough to eat. In most high-income countries, government programs exist to support pregnant and breastfeeding women. In addition, many community churches and civic groups operate food pantries where we can refer those experiencing food insecurity. We need to have lists of these local resources available to hand out as needed.

When serving in low-resource areas, it's important to build food distribution into your budget during pregnancy care. At Mercy In Action clinics, we identify malnourished women early in pregnancy with low mid-upper arm circumference (MUAC) measurements. If a woman's MUAC score indicates danger, we don't just take note; we take action. She leaves each prenatal visit with food, freely given and offered with dignity, because in places where resources are scarce, nourishment is considered a form of medical care during pregnancy.

We are currently taking care of a young mother named Tracie who was diagnosed recently with tuberculosis (TB). Tracie weighs 29.5 kilograms (65 pounds), and the tape measure on her upper arm shows a MUAC reading in the red danger zone. While helping her access TB medication, I told our team that we also needed to supplement her food. I reminded our team of how Paul Farmer's TB DOTS program emphasized not just delivering medication, but ensuring patients had the support, both nutritional and relational, to complete treatment.

One of the Imago Dei Health & Birth Center staff suggested coordinating with a nearby store to deliver the food to her, with us covering the cost. Marlene, the head midwife, spoke right up and respectfully disagreed with that approach. She said, "While I understand the concern about the transportation expenses, it doesn't sit right with me. We are not simply giving food to address Tracie's malnutrition;

we want her to feel honored, valued, and loved. I believe our presence plays a significant role in that, especially during this time, which must be very difficult for her."

Marlene told me later that she remembered my story about King's Table, and that is why she had to say something. The concept had taken root; she knew our care must never prioritize efficiency at the cost of presence.

EXPRESSIONS OF CARE

Personally, I like to feed people homemade food as an expression of caring whenever possible. Baking a small birthday cake for the twenty-four-hour postpartum visit can elevate the sense of hospitality, as can bringing a basket of muffins to share. I've been told by family and friends that baking seems to be one of my love languages. Perhaps that is why I can't resist watching *The Great British Bake Off* whenever I get the chance!

Serving homemade snacks at childbirth classes is one way to model healthy eating during pregnancy. Similarly, serving something delicious and hot out of the oven during the morning break of an intense midwifery seminar eases the tension of learning resuscitation or hemorrhage management. I have also baked and carried many a loaf of fresh, hot bread wrapped in a new kitchen towel to a family grieving a pregnancy loss, or just in need of a little extra nurturing and comfort for whatever reason.

Susan, one of our graduates, told me she brings a grocery bag full of fresh vegetables with her to home births. While the client is in early labor, she steps into the kitchen and makes a pot of soup for after the birth. That is the kind of thing that will stick with a family forever. She's a servant leader with her sleeves rolled up, ladling broth into bowls between postpartum vital sign checks.

Jenny Fox, a member of our staff, told me she has seen firsthand that food does not need to be homemade to show sincere hospitality. She shared with me that during a recent long home-birth labor, friends brought a ready-made meal and simple, store-bought snacks just when everyone's energy was flagging. My late husband used to buy pizza to bring down to the birth center for all the midwives if a labor interrupted dinnertime. The midwives in the Philippines still talk about that, remembering fondly how he also brought them boxes of candy on Valentine's Day and other holidays.

Hospitality lives in the heart and can be expressed by everyone, regardless of natural talent. While some may offer hospitality through food, others share it through listening, service, or simply being present. True hospitality is not limited by ability but by willingness.

Daily, I find myself inspired anew by the creative work we do as midwives and the opportunities we have to change people's lives with simple, meaningful acts. Our Mercy In Action leaders often say to each other, "It's not just about meeting expectations, it's about trying to exceed them." What kind of transformation would happen if we regularly gave people more than they expect? Not in a flashy, superficial way, but in a deeply thoughtful, human way. Allowing hospitality to saturate our care until the experience itself becomes a kind of healing to the spirit of the people we serve.

That's the transformation I want to see in maternal and child healthcare everywhere in the world. That would assuredly shift outcomes, and more mothers and babies would thrive under that system of care if it were available and affordable to them.

UNREASONABLE HOSPITALITY

While I was walking through the library recently, a book caught my attention. The title was *Unreasonable Hospitality*. In this captivating book, Will Guidara argues that the concept of unreasonable hospitality is applicable to any business and should not be limited to for-profit service establishments like Michelin-starred restaurants or high-end hotels. I completely agree, and appreciate his use of the phrase "unreasonable hospitality," by which he essentially means being willing to invest extra effort and care to create unforgettable experiences and build lasting relationships. Guidara argues that achieving extraordinary success in any field often requires an unreasonable pursuit of excellence and a commitment to hospitality. We should all be as dedicated to making people feel great as we are to our core product or service.

Applying this to our midwifery strategy, I would say that unreasonable hospitality should not be reserved only for pregnant women who can afford private midwifery fees. Rather, hospitality that is unreasonable for its generosity should be present in all our prenatal exam rooms, birth centers, and hospitals worldwide. What a different world that would be.

HOMEFULNESS

Then there is an even deeper hospitality that occurs in the spaces we create for people to enter into our presence. It's known in some religious circles as *homefulness*. Holistic care at its best, the concept of homefulness has been identified as a comprehensive sense of belonging that encompasses body, soul, and spirit. Making people feel welcome in our presence is a central aspect of this form of hospitality. From ancient prophets to the words of Jesus, welcoming strangers and aliens is encouraged as an age-old practice that is about extending genuine care and creating a sense of belonging, reflecting God's welcoming nature.

Homefulness extends beyond the places we invite people into on our terms, making hospitality an option everywhere, without boundaries. It means bringing a healing presence into every space with us. In its fullest sense, it is to become someone with whom others can feel at home. The belief is that home is created through loving relationships and not merely through owning or occupying a building. The best midwives carry homefulness with them, making others feel at ease in their presence by treating them as having great value.

We need to press into this concept within midwifery. Because homefulness doesn't depend on location, it is the intentional focus on helping others feel a sense of welcome and worth in our presence. In a time when loneliness has reached epidemic levels, and the temptation to reduce problems to "us versus them" narratives is rampant, the simple but profound gift of belonging has never been more needed. Birth care at its best can offer that sense of belonging. Not just to clients and patients, but to students, other birth workers like doulas, and colleagues in other medical professions alike. If we create a culture of homefulness, we then have the opportunity to invite those around us to come into a safe and respectful place.

DIFFERENT EXPRESSIONS

Over the years, hospitality has taken on many forms for me, always shaped by the needs I see around me. Early in my career in Alaska, it meant welcoming a homeless pregnant teenager to sleep on our couch while I searched for a safe place for her to stay long-term. For Scott and me, that early instinct to open our home, and our lives, became a thread through our forty-four years of marriage. Whether it was inviting someone in for a few nights or sharing community living spaces in various parts of the world, we found that true hospitality begins at home, and sometimes, it means giving someone outside your family a place at your table, or a key to the front door. Even now, as a widow, I carry this tradition on.

HOSPITALITY TO STUDENTS

In our midwifery school environment, hospitality means furnishing the spaces with warmth and intention. I remember once, while setting up for a new semester, I made plans to remove a worn-looking rocking chair from the dorm because I thought it was too shabby to keep. But as I arrived with two men to carry it out, a new student who had arrived early was sitting in that very chair. Her reaction to our attempt to remove it was surprisingly vehement, so I backed off. Later I learned she had just endured a profound personal loss, and somehow that old chair had become a small source of comfort in an unfamiliar setting. So, the ratty chair stayed until she left campus, because it was where she always sat. That, too, was hospitality.

Anxiety and fear are normal during the pre-service midwife journey at times, and especially vulnerable is the time when students seek out a preceptor and begin a clinical apprenticeship. Memories from my early days as a student midwife—when I was the one feeling scared and unsure—are forever colored positively, despite the unsettling twists and turns I encountered, because of the way I was welcomed by my preceptors with boundless hospitality.

LEAVING ALASKA

In early 1983, my husband and I made the monumental decision to leave our home in Alaska temporarily so I could study midwifery. We arranged a move to New Mexico, as it was one of only a handful of states at that time that recognized and licensed direct-entry midwives. Having no money to pay for my education, we sold most everything we owned before taking the long flight with our three-year-old son, heading bravely into the unknown to pursue a vision.

That is how I arrived in the Southwest as a stranger, having arranged an apprenticeship before leaving Alaska. I was hungry to soak up every ounce of learning I could in order to become the best midwife I could possibly be. Our hope was that the money from selling our possessions would last until I could meet the requirements to get a New Mexico license. Midwives in Alaska were depending on me to return not only with a license for credibility but also with the knowledge needed to attempt to pass legislation to get midwives recognized in our state.

My first stop upon arriving in the Lower 48 was a midwife conference. It was there that I discovered quite by accident that the midwife who had agreed through correspondence to be my preceptor was not qualified (this was before the days of the Internet, when verifying someone's credentials was not easy to do the way it is now). Through a brief encounter with the maternal director for the state of New Mexico at the conference, I found out this person was in process but did not yet have a license to practice midwifery.

You can probably imagine the desperate feelings of panic that coursed through me upon learning this unfortunate news. In that moment, I was sure that I had bankrupted our family by chasing a dream that now could not happen. I cried myself to sleep that night.

The following morning at the conference, a small miracle of sorts occurred when the maternal director, obviously having taken pity on me, introduced me to Elizabeth Gilmore and her then-midwifery partner, Tish Demmin. They listened as I told of traveling all the way from Alaska and now having no preceptor because of the deception. Elizabeth and Tish went off to confer together briefly before coming back and announcing that they had decided to take a chance on me. I was offered an apprenticeship in Taos on the spot, a coveted position, it turned out. And my life was changed forever by that decision.

What awaited our family in Taos was something I hadn't expected, given the last-minute nature of my arrival as a stranger. The midwives at the Northern New Mexico Midwifery Center gave our family a warm welcome that wildly exceeded my almost nonexistent expectations. Elizabeth introduced me to clients in a way that was so warm and respectful that I was immediately accepted by them. The midwives invited me to lunch with them on clinic days and encouraged me to share my thoughts and opinions during discussions around the table. I was welcomed without reservation into their inner professional midwifery circle, and integrated so thoroughly that I flourished as an apprentice, meeting all my licensure requirements in less time than expected.

And it wasn't just business. Elizabeth exuded a sense of homefulness in her very being. She and her husband Carl invited Scott and me into their home. Our children played together, and they often brought us on fun adventures with them, hiking to hot springs or attending cultural events.

This welcome, this unexpected hospitality, impacted me deeply, and laid a foundation that has shaped my life as a midwife and midwifery educator. The generosity I experienced helped me become the kind of leader I am now, one who remembers how much it builds confidence to be welcomed into a space with people you look up to. The midwives in Taos, with their open hearts and skillful teaching, set the stage for powerful learning in my life. The birth center provided the fertile garden soil for me to grow and bloom, but it was the hospitality of the midwives that was my sun and rain.

Elizabeth eventually became much more than just my preceptor; she became my trusted mentor, close friend, and collaborator in providing midwifery education for the next thirty years. When she died, I was asked to give the eulogy at her funeral, and I wrote a tribute to her that was published in *Midwifery Today* magazine. Thus closed a chapter on a treasured friendship with one of the most generous, visionary, and hospitable people I have ever known.

PRACTICAL HOSPITALITY

In my years living in the Philippines, hospitality has often looked like meeting basic survival needs of those around us, such as rebuilding a roof after a storm or making an unlivable space safe again. My son Sean, who would later become a Harvard-trained doctor, remembers his first introduction to the social determinants of health. A young child in the feeding program he oversaw in the Philippines was diagnosed with severe intestinal worms, and Sean discovered that the child's family was living underground in a cave-like dugout. After treating the child and his family with albendazole, he and a team of workers from our clinic dug into the contaminated dirt to lay proper flooring so that the child could be healthy.

During the global pandemic, hospitality looked like loading our ambulance with food bags and delivering them door-to-door to families who were on lockdown without food and unable to earn a living. Ambulances were the only vehicles allowed on the road in those early months of 2020, so we made good use of our mobility to get to families who were shut in. Later, each birth center set up free food pantries that we kept stocked until people could work again.

At times, a spirit of hospitality necessitates intentionally prioritizing the needs of an individual experiencing poverty or vulnerability when making decisions about resources and care. This preferential perspective acknowledges that individuals with fewer resources often face greater barriers and deserve targeted support to ensure their basic needs are met. Hospitality respects human dignity.

Hospitality toward the most vulnerable also affirms that the well-being of the whole community is deeply connected to how we care for its most vulnerable members. It has been said that what harms women and children today will harm society as a whole tomorrow, and the opposite is also true. When a community prioritizes care for a mother facing poverty by ensuring access to housing, food, and reliable support, her children are more likely to thrive, pressure on social services is reduced, and overall community stability is strengthened. In this way, care for the most vulnerable sustains the well-being of all.

SERVICE AT HOME

At home births, in addition to the actual midwifery care, I have a habit of starting the laundry and washing the dishes before I leave the home after the birth. No one asks me to do this, and no one really expects me to, but that's what makes it hospitality. It's not just about welcoming families into our own space, such as a birth center or hospital, but also how we enter someone else's sacred space with attention and intention. Home births offer us the opportunity to serve in ways that make people feel truly valued and nurtured. Often, it is our going above and beyond that makes all the difference.

Hospitality can be offered anywhere, and is often something small: offering a postpartum mother a steaming cup of her favorite tea, prepared just the way she likes it with cream and honey. Remembering the names of her older children. At its heart, hospitality means tuning in, paying attention, and quietly meeting needs before they're even spoken. It is a beautiful form of nurturing.

BIRTH CENTER HOSPITALITY

In 2015, Mercy In Action purchased a building in Boise to establish Mercy Birth Center, a pilot project. My daughter-in-law Rose, a midwife, started and ran this nonprofit birth center as an arm of Mercy In Action. In this open access birth model, we centered care around access for low-income women, removing barriers at the door and placing a high value on service and hospitality.

The goal of this birth center was to reach families overlooked and without access to care who were falling through the cracks. The birth center provided care for refugees, pregnant teenagers, those recently released from incarceration, those without a reliable income, and anyone else who was seeking midwifery care. It was a true open-access model, as I had done decades before in Fairbanks, Alaska.

A large percentage of the clients who entered the Boise birth center were living below the poverty line and on government assistance, and for the rest, we utilized a sliding scale based on income and family size. We never charged for anything on top of their Medicaid or private insurance, and we never asked for payment up front for the first visit. One mother told us she was undocumented, so that became a pro bono case.

Whether they came early or late to care, the midwives would take a history and do risk screening before conducting a full prenatal exam, and then determine how to best help the pregnancy and birth to be as safe as possible. If the woman qualified for assistance, the midwives helped her fill out paperwork, because navigating the system is often difficult. Our dedicated staff shared the same belief that a maternity healthcare system should be responsive and welcoming, built around quality care for everyone, not just those who have the means to pay. We proved that it is absolutely possible to make this open-access model work anywhere; it just takes creativity and imagination.

For the time this model birth center was open in Boise, clients said it was the little things that really added up to make it a special experience. The waiting room was cozy and beautifully decorated with birth art, and each exam room featured a love seat and a small set of toys, so the couples would feel welcome and children could join their mother without getting bored. Rose set up a lovely tea station, always stocked with a pleasing variety of teas, pretty mugs, and honey sticks. It quickly became part of the birth center's culture to be welcomed in and guided straight to that corner of comfort to make a fresh, hot cup of something soothing before beginning the exam.

If someone arrived on the city bus, Rose would drive them home after their appointment, and then arrange to come to their home for the next checkup if transportation was a problem. Childbirth classes were free to the entire community, regardless of where the attendees planned to give birth, and delicious-yet-healthy homemade snacks were served alongside the informative and interactive teaching by the midwives.

As a final personalized touch, Rose knit a bespoke baby hat for each infant born in her care, often working on it during the quiet hours of early labor while watchfully monitoring progress. This simple gesture was priceless in how it made families feel; they knew that love was being woven into every stitch, crafted especially for their child.

THE MODEL WORKS

Before we opened our Boise, Idaho, model birth center, I would sometimes hear comments during our seminars in America along the lines of, "What you do in the Philippines wouldn't work here in American midwifery." I'd gently explain that this model wasn't new to me, that I had practiced it for thirteen years in Alaska at the start of my career, long before our international work began. Still, some would dismiss it with a shrug and say, "Well, that was a long time ago."

Our birth center in Boise from 2015 to 2019 demonstrated that an open access birth center in America was still possible, feasible, viable, and desirable. We were glad to find that our model birth center did prove again what is possible in an urban, highly industrialized setting, but that was not the main motivation. Rose wanted to love and care for the people in her community, and she represented Mercy In Action well in doing so for the years it was open.

UNDER A TREE

Once during those years living in Boise, Rose encountered a couple seeking shelter from the sun under a tree in the Walmart parking lot. Her midwife's eye noted that the woman seemed to be in labor. Rose called me, as I was in the States at the time, and we agreed on a plan to help this young couple who had run out of gas on a road trip and had nowhere to turn when labor began. They had intended to be in California before the baby arrived.

Rose and Ian offered their home for the birth, but while monitoring the labor, we noted mild hypertension with clonus, and determined that early signs of preeclampsia ruled out the home birth this first-time mother desired. We got her a referral with an accommodating doctor, and Jen, a midwifery student who had coincidentally met them the weekend before at a campground, accompanied them to the hospital and stayed until she gave birth.

The next day, these young parents called me, scared, because a discharge nurse was threatening to call child protective services since they could not provide a physical address. I talked to the nurse and gave her my address, assuring her I would give them a place to live for the next few days, and told her that as midwives, Rose and I were prepared to provide free postpartum monitoring. A few of Rose's former birth clients, hearing of the need, stepped up with a car seat and baby clothes, and we purchased other items they needed. When they climbed back into their van to complete their journey to the Pacific Ocean, breastfeeding was well-established, the mother was healthy, and the parents were reveling in the afterglow of a positive birth experience.

This situation could have easily turned out with a very different outcome. Generous hospitality, given beyond reason and without charge at their moment of greatest need, provided this young family with everything they needed to be safe, both physically and emotionally. Whether in clinic spaces, a home, or under a tree in a parking lot, our goal is to invite pregnant women into a space of care that communicates hospitality from the very first encounter.

KNITTING HOSPITALITY

Just as Rose knit blessings into every little hat she made while running our birth center in America, volunteers around the world have joined in, creating handmade hats for Mercy In Action babies born in the Philippines. There's just something about being given a brand-new baby hat that makes the parents feel their baby is special and valued. The time, the care, the thought that goes into each stitch —it carries meaning beyond the obvious warmth. It's an enduring act of thoughtful hospitality.

Giving a newborn-size hat to each baby born in our centers started when we only needed twenty-five handmade hats a month, and at the time that felt manageable. But when the number of babies being born each month climbed, reaching over one hundred births per month at one point, we wondered if we could keep it up. We believed it was worth the effort because these little hats had come to mean so much to the parents. The hats were especially meaningful to families who carried the weight of generational poverty and rarely received anything new, much less something handcrafted just for them. So we launched the Mercy In Action baby hat project with a simple invitation to our families and donors: If you can knit or crochet or use a simple loom, please help us make sure every baby is welcomed with a hat made by hand.

Thousands of hats have materialized over the years. They arrive at our headquarters or directly at the Philippine birth centers from longtime faithful supporters, from mothers and children knitting side by side, from knitting circles organized around church groups. In making baby hats, our former clients and our team's families have been particularly generous. Our oldest knitter is in her nineties, and we have had children making hats on looms beginning as young as six years old. All want to take part in this tender expression of welcome to Mercy In Action babies, whom they will probably never meet.

In our birth centers, this simple gesture, giving each baby a new handmade baby hat, says louder than words that we value them. New parents, many who have no other new clothes for this child, feel the love. The hats embody the spirit of hospitality in tangible form. Parents tell us that people in the community often point and say, "Mercy baby!" when they see the hat. In the end, the hat isn't just for the baby. It's a message to the parents and to the wider community that they are not alone. These children will be lovingly watched over. The hat is more than a gift. It has become a symbol of the larger hospitality that welcomes and surrounds each new member of the community.

Years after our baby hat project launched and was going strong, I came across a study on newborn mortality and morbidity in low- and middle-income countries. Many of the best solutions in this study were surprisingly low-tech, with one of the key interventions highlighted being the simple newborn hat, which helps prevent cold stress by keeping babies' body heat from dissipating too quickly after birth and in the days and weeks that follow. Since the head is where babies lose the most heat, a hat can mean the difference between thriving and struggling, even between life and death.

When I read that, I had an epiphany about the connection between hospitality and evidence-based interventions in neonatal complications and death. It was encouraging to know that what we were already doing in our little birth centers was being affirmed on a global scale—one tiny hat at a time.

HOSPITALITY AS THE NORM

Unfortunately, such hospitality is not the norm in healthcare. That's why we may need to break a few old rules to change the culture. Some of the rigid systems we've inherited in healthcare were designed more for efficiency than compassion, more for profit than achieving great outcomes. If how we make someone feel matters, along with all the other things we do, we may need to rethink how health and wellness occur. Maybe the act of hospitality has the power to bring healing, security, and comfort in a way that nothing else can.

When I describe extending this kind of abundant hospitality, there are always going to be a few people who criticize the concept, finding it unreasonable and undeserved. But the women and families who receive it? They don't criticize or find fault. They are honored by the attention and deeply grateful for the care. They tell others about the wonderful birth care they received. The families we serve in this manner will remember not only the quality maternity care, but also how they were made to feel. The boost of value we bestow through abundant hospitality just may be a game changer in how well a mother or couple can cope with the stress of pregnancy, the pain of labor, and the exhausting early days of parenting. It ties to a strategy for improving outcomes.

CRITICAL CARE HOSPITALITY

Critical care hospitality extends into the medical realm and encompasses a level of service necessary to support a person through a maternity care crisis. This is how we respond to the deeper physical and emotional needs that can arise during unplanned and sometimes tragic events in maternity care.

When someone calls experiencing a miscarriage or has not felt their baby kick in a few hours, one of us on the midwife call team goes to them immediately, even in the middle of the night. We don't charge extra for that. And if a mother needs more postpartum visits than usual, because she or the baby is not thriving, those extra visits are given at no additional cost. We work hard to ensure that extra care is not perceived as inconvenient or too expensive to afford.

Critical care hospitality is clinical care offered with a readiness to adapt when a client's needs fall outside the routine. I've made home visits for weeks to give prenatal care to a woman in bed threatened with preterm labor. I've made daily house calls to check someone's blood pressure near the end of pregnancy when preeclampsia signs were creeping in. That kind of vigilant monitoring comes from knowing our purpose is to help people safely through danger. Critical care hospitality such as this will move the odds in favor of a good outcome during a high-risk pregnancy.

Some providers charge for individual visits and emergency treatments, but we suggest that, if care can't be free, it be based on a predetermined global fee, as it better aligns with our values and removes barriers to care. If a family knows they will be charged more for follow-up or extra visits, they may forgo that care to save money, and thus miss out on midwifery care at a point when it is most crucial. In all our birth centers, we accept what insurance pays without additional cash charges, so as not to put an additional burden on the family. It is of note that free maternity care or an affordable and transparent fee, with no add-ons for complications, is considered the global best-practice standard.

HOSPITALITY HONORS CULTURE

Hospitality in midwifery is about creating a space where every person feels respected, and where who they are and where they are from is not just tolerated, but honored.

On a trip to study birth customs in Ecuador, I once met a community of women in the highlands who refused to go to the hospital to give birth. I learned this was in part because their tradition is to squat during labor, wearing their wide skirts to keep their modesty intact, and this behavior was not allowed in hospitals. Instead, the hospital staff required them to remove the large, colorful skirts that were part of their cultural identity and put on a flimsy hospital gown. These thin, short gowns, open in the back, were considered by these women to be an affront to their sense of dignity, something they found shameful to wear. Being forced to remove their ethnic clothing and give birth lying down and exposed felt deeply disrespectful to them. So when labor began, they would stay home without a skilled attendant to assist them at the time of birth. And some of them suffered for it when birth complications occurred. Some of their babies died needlessly; mortality was much higher among this people group than in the rest of Ecuador.

I wondered how many lives have been lost over the simple matter of clothing and mandated birth position. How easily a more hospitable environment in that nation's hospitals could have saved lives. It wouldn't have cost anything to let them keep their skirts on and squat. Imagine if the hospital staff had said, instead, "We will work around your traditions, respecting your choice of clothes and posture, to keep you and your baby safe in the event of childbirth complications or emergencies."

Cultural humility is not an add-on to care. It's a vital part of hospitality. If people do not feel safe and respected, they may not seek help during a problem or engage with health care providers at all. And if they don't trust us enough to seek our help, we have no chance to impact outcomes. True hospitality pays attention to culture. It adapts and welcomes, and that welcome may be the difference between life and death.

MATERNITY WAITING HOMES

At one time in our history, one of our hospitality projects involved building a small group of maternity waiting homes for women from surrounding tribal villages. The World Health Organization (WHO) identified maternity waiting homes as a key strategy to "bridge the geographical gap" in obstetric care for rural women. By providing women with a safe and welcoming place to stay near medical care as they approached delivery, these homes helped create better outcomes for both mothers and babies.

Rose had the vision to apply for a grant through One Day's Wages to make these homes possible, and they became a meaningful addition to the care and support we were able to offer our community. For us, this project beautifully tied hospitality to improving birth outcomes.

We chose a piece of land on a mountainside near our birth center, located where the footpath descending from the mountains naturally passed. This allowed tribal women to come down ahead of labor and wait nearby, rather than attempting a long and often dangerous journey down the mountain once labor had begun, as the trail was steep, rocky, and crossed a river at several different points. The homes were built using nipa and thatched roofing, in a style familiar to the Aeta people. At the same time, the homes included electricity, and a building with bathrooms and shower facilities was on-site, offering safety and comfort while remaining culturally familiar.

The value of these maternity waiting homes became especially clear over time. When we identified a severely malnourished pregnant woman in her eighth month, she moved into one of the homes so we could provide three nourishing meals each day and closely support her health while waiting for labor to begin. At other times, women who gave birth during the rainy season stayed with us when the river was too high to cross safely. They remained in the waiting homes until the water receded enough for them to return to their mountain villages. In these moments, the maternity waiting homes served not only as shelter, but as places of protection and hospitality during a vulnerable season of life.

THE RIPPLE EFFECT OF HOSPITALITY

Abundant hospitality isn't just words. It is a value we hold dear. When midwives embody hospitality in how we lead, how we relate, and how we engage with those around us, it changes the culture. Hospitality is an integral part of our mode of operation in all the clinics Mercy In Action builds and sponsors. We are intentionally creating a culture of generosity, of welcome, of service that catches on and spreads outward.

No matter the outcome of their story, it will almost certainly be better for every pregnant woman and her baby because healthcare providers were kind, concerned, and welcoming. The same is true for students entering into an apprenticeship with us; it's a vulnerable season, as many seasoned midwives can remember and personally attest to. People never forget how you made them feel, even after they've forgotten the details of what you said or did.

UNIQUELY POSITIONED

For our clients and patients, for our students, for the broader community of healthcare providers, and for one another, midwives are uniquely positioned to embody hospitality. The remarkable power of giving people more than they expect or feel they deserve fits perfectly with my belief that midwifery is not just a clinical profession but a relational calling. The side benefit is that it makes our job more creative and therefore more fun and enjoyable. If we are enjoying our work, it is more likely to be sustainable over the years.

For those midwives who are already doing too much, hospitality might feel like one more thing on an already full plate. But once you catch the spirit of abundant hospitality and take ownership of it, something shifts. It becomes life-giving and joyful to dream up new ways to bless others. Try it. It might help you get priorities better aligned, and you may just find a fresh sense of energy and delight awakening within you. Inspiration is everywhere.

An added blessing is that this kind of care nourishes both the giver and the receiver. Our midwives often share that after joining Mercy In Action and learning to extend the same respect and hospitality in the clinic that they would extend in their own homes, they experienced a profound sense of fulfillment and job satisfaction.

THE BLESSING OF A STRANGER

In our Philippines birth centers, the first thing someone entering sees is a dispenser of clean, cold water. These drink stations are intentional. In places where even water is bought and sold for prices the poor cannot easily afford, this is a small act that says, "Everyone is welcome here." That first offering of cold water may be the gentlest way to break the ice, but what it communicates sets the scene for the trustworthy maternity care that will follow.

I find that we will naturally become more hospitable to those around us as we cultivate a sense of purpose and vocation, and work on building a strong character. I believe that the intangible concepts we have been exploring so far in this book are the very things that change outcomes and, on a larger scale, could cause ripples of profound change in how maternity healthcare is delivered. We can all choose to be leaders in the way forward. Hospitality is a beautiful form of servant leadership, a topic we will explore in the next chapter.

As we conclude this chapter, I would like to issue a challenge. You may not have previously thought that washing the mountain of dishes in the sink at a home birth was your job, but what if you rolled up your sleeves? You may have assumed that basic communication skills are all it takes for a birth team to function at its best, but what if something as simple as sharing occasional meals together could deepen that bond and connect you even more? Midwifery businesses need to cover expenses, but is there room in your model for a bit of pro bono or barter? Could you find a creative way to offer the first prenatal checkup without barriers? To simply listen, evaluate, and respond with compassion before asking for up-front payment? Could you erase the debt for a family who experienced a pregnancy loss? Ask yourself, can we measure the difference in outcomes that these small changes might make?

An old-world Celtic blessing inspires us to think of how the blessing of hospitality often rebounds to the giver:

> *Seeing a stranger approach,*
> *I would put food in the eating place*
> *drink in the drinking place*
> *music in the listening place,*
> *and look with joy for the blessing of God,*
> *who often comes to my home*
> *in the blessing of a stranger.*
>
> — TRADITIONAL CELTIC BLESSING

PAUSE FOR REFLECTION

If hospitality were treated as essential to healing rather than optional, how would your daily practice look different? What is one specific change you could begin this week to help patients or families feel more seen, heard, and cared for? Where in your setting would this shift create the greatest impact for both patient experience and team culture?

4
UPSIDE-DOWN LEADERSHIP

The key to successful leadership is influence, not authority.

— KEN BLANCHARD

MY GOAL WAS NEVER LEADERSHIP. IT WAS TO EASE SUFFERING. I accepted leadership roles to reach that goal. I have seen the same pattern in many others. They weren't seeking leadership, but they stepped into a gap to meet a need. In this chapter, I will share with you some stories related to leadership and some of the key principles I have learned over the years. It can be summarized by the *why*, the *who*, and the *how*. In the context of my life's work, the *why* is to improve the health and life of mothers and babies around the world. The *who* is those who are leaders in birth work and speaks to their identity, personalities, and character. And the *how* is through setting an example. This would involve things like servant leadership, cultivating more midwives and advocates, working as a team, finding creative solutions to complex problems, and persevering through challenges.

JOURNEY INTO ACCIDENTAL LEADERSHIP

Here is how it started for me: My husband, Scott, and I were living in Alaska, building an off-grid cabin in the woods with our own hands. Newly married and planning our family, we already knew we wanted to have a home birth when the time came. I had never met anyone who had a home birth, and there were no midwives in my area, so it took quite an effort to make it happen. Looking back, I realize it also took leadership skills to plan the safe and respectful birth I wanted for my own babies.

As a child and teen, I found myself frequently listening to the birth stories of other women, many of them riddled with trauma. I couldn't shake the feeling that all the suffering was unnecessary. Then one day, with a sense of awe but not surprise, I realized that my interest in birth had grown into a calling to become a midwife.

Shortly after our first son was born, I stepped into the birth world, attending the births of friends and helping out where I could. Eventually I reached a point where I knew I needed to commit fully and pursue a solid education to become a licensed midwife. Scott and I sold nearly everything we owned to fund my training. There were no educational opportunities available in Alaska at that time, so we headed to New Mexico with our toddler in tow. Upon my return to Alaska, I quickly became a cofounder of the Midwives Association of Alaska and spearheaded the effort to pass legislation recognizing and licensing direct-entry midwives. And just like that, my journey into leadership began.

I was only twenty-four when I found myself borrowing a skirt and blazer from my friend Michele and flying to the state capital to testify. A judge had ruled that delivering babies constituted the practice of medicine in Alaska, and if we did not pass a midwifery bill during the current legislative session, it would become illegal for any of us to attend births.

In Juneau, I testified before Senate and House committees, and I quoted statistics on the safety and effectiveness of the midwifery profession to dozens of individual legislators as well, my heart pounding every time. I had never spoken to power like that before, let alone tried to influence legislation. It was a steep learning curve. But I did it because I believed families deserved to have a choice about home birth, and midwives were the only providers offering that choice.

Back home in Fairbanks, I appeared on TV and radio shows and was interviewed for the nightly news. I rallied support from parents and taught them how to write letters and testify. In May 1985, on the last day of the session, our midwifery bill passed with overwhelming support in both the House and Senate. A week later, Governor Sheffield invited me to stand beside him as he signed the midwifery bill into law. With heartfelt congratulations, he handed me the pen he used to sign the bill, and that moment was photographed and featured in newspapers across the state.

It would still take me years to use the word *leader* for myself. However, I've come to see that leadership is rarely something we declare. It's something we grow into, one brave act at a time. At some point, we begin to understand that leadership happens in the space between a need arising and our realizing the moment calls for us to step forward and meet it.

If you'd asked me before my first pregnancy in 1979 if I thought of myself as a leader, I would have answered no, definitely not. I am a bit shy by nature. But now I have been leading for so long I could not tell you the exact moment when I accepted the title of leader. I just found over the years that as I wanted things to happen, and started moving in that direction, others followed. As it turns out, this is often how leadership begins, not with a title but rather with a simple willingness to serve. I have now been a leader for almost five decades and have studied the topic of leadership almost as long. I recently earned a doctorate in a program named Creative Leadership. But for a servant leader, credentials are not about privilege or status but about the capacity to serve.

WHO IS A LEADER?

Leadership has been described as *the ability to influence another person's thinking, behavior, or development.* By that definition, most healthcare workers, and certainly anyone who is a teacher or a parent, is already leading. We may not all carry titles or hold authority, but we all have influence, and that influence can significantly impact birth outcomes.

Leadership isn't always obvious to the casual observer. Sometimes a leader is just somebody willing to step up or go first, not because they are the most confident but because the work matters to them. No one is ever too young to lead, just as no one is ever too old to lead. Pay attention, and you may see leadership happening in many unexpected places.

If you want to make a difference in this work, you will find yourself doing the work of leadership. All birth workers will find themselves teaching and leading, at least one-on-one, and midwives must learn the basics of leading so they can excel at providing care. For those midwives who are or will be preceptors to a student or younger midwife at some point, that is leadership too. So it is important to be a lifelong learner and keep growing in leadership.

PERSONALITIES

There are some misleading stereotypes about leadership. It's not about being the loudest voice in the room, and it does not require being extroverted, arrogant, or unshakably confident. Some of the most high-impact leaders I've known are quiet, steady people with a deep well of conviction and faith in their cause. Leaders come with all types of personalities. But all the best leaders I know have two things in common: They have a servant's heart, and they lead by example. This means they have done the internal work, because having this capacity to prefer others over ourselves often means pursuing our own emotional wholeness first.

THE INNER AND OUTER JOURNEY

In previous chapters we have discussed several factors that lead to good birth outcomes, such as adopting a moral purpose, developing character, and offering genuine hospitality with love. Now let's add humble, hopeful leadership. I have read that teams can only grow as deep and wide as the inner work a leader has done. We lead best when we know who we are, have faced our own faults with honesty, and allowed hardship to refine our character, all the while holding fast to a vision of a better world. Servant leaders must begin with an inner journey and come to know themselves well so that they are ready to lead with humility. Those who aspire to lead should first learn to lead themselves. Until you can master your inner self, you cannot serve others well.

However, to make a lasting impact, we can't stay in our heads and hearts alone. We also need an outward journey where we put our hands to work to bring ideas to life, devise creative solutions, and follow through on the purpose that drives us. This outward journey is where we execute ideas and put well-researched best practices at the forefront to improve the lives of those we serve. Let's look at a few keys to leading effectively.

LEADERS SET THE TONE

I believe lasting transformation begins with people who are thriving. As leaders, we set the tone for whether good or bad vibes flow through our teams. When we model generosity and hospitality, our teams grow and flourish. Midwives and students who feel valued will reflect that same value back to the families they serve. The same holds true whether it is on-call or shift work; the leaders shape the culture of a shift or a birth, so let it be marked by warmth, attentiveness, and welcome to the workers as well as to the clients and patients.

How we relate to allied healthcare professionals matters too, especially during and after transfers of care. A simple gesture of gratitude after a home-to-hospital transfer can build goodwill, ease tension, and pave the way for better collaboration the next time. Strong relationships across the healthcare system improve outcomes, but someone has to take the lead in opening those channels, and that someone might be you.

The way we treat our team should mirror how we hope they treat clients and patients: with kindness, encouragement, and respect. If we want that to happen, we'd better be aware of the power of behavior modeling. Good leaders should share the load, notice when someone needs support, and create a culture of appreciation. And while the work we do is serious, we are allowed to laugh and have fun too. A joyful, secure team of people is a resilient team. That joy is part of what binds us and bonds us to one another. Because when a team feels well-loved and well-led, it creates a kind of synergy that gets things done in a way no one person could do by themselves. Together we are stronger than any one of us alone.

THE INVERTED PYRAMID

The best leaders do not seek a position for themselves; they serve others. They invest generously in developing and empowering new leaders, multiplying their influence far beyond what they could accomplish without help. Leadership is rarely comfortable, but it is profoundly rewarding. It is especially meaningful when it creates lasting change in birth culture, benefiting generations to come.

Servant leadership is an upside-down approach to leadership because it is not about traditional structures of power and hierarchy. It is an intentional choice to lead from a place of serving rather than a bossy place of control. The best leadership begins with humility and the desire to lift others up. Servant leadership that nurtures those we are responsible for and raises up future leaders is both a spiritual posture and a practical strategy.

Midwifery, with its model based on shared decision-making and informed consent, works best with a mentoring approach. We are in the business of promoting healthy behavior and creating an environment that enables the development of knowledgeable, confident, and loving families. Midwifery education traditionally includes at least two years of apprenticeship, a time-honored, structured, hands-on journey of learning by doing, side by side with those who have walked this path before. Clinical skills are developed through observation, supervised practice, and gradually taking on more responsibility under the steady guidance of a seasoned practitioner. All this is leadership.

Leadership of our individual birth teams and local, state, national, and international midwifery organizations can also thrive in a model where the traditional hierarchy is flipped and leaders exist to serve, empower, and remove obstacles in the way of fostering growth and development toward better birth outcomes.

You may see yourself as only a mildly influential leader within birth work, or you may be a recognized leader with a title. Regardless of your status, you will need to use your influence to serve well if you want to help improve birth outcomes. This concept of wholehearted servant leadership is one of the secrets of our success in achieving the good outcomes that Mercy In Action birth centers have enjoyed for decades.

Servant leadership flips the usual picture of power. It's not about being at the top; it's about holding up the foundation. Imagine a pyramid. In traditional leadership, the leader sits at the top, and the people below support their goals. But servant leaders turn that structure upside-down. The leader places themselves at the bottom, not a position meant to diminish their role, but to serve the mission better and to achieve the most return on effort, which can only be accomplished with a team.

HELPERS AND HEROES

Midwifery has always made the best sense to me through this servant leadership lens. We don't walk into the room as the boss; we come in as the helper. We are the experts in the room present to support the well-being of the mother and baby. We kneel. We listen. We share decision-making with the family gathered. As leaders, whether we are running a birth practice, educating parents, or mentoring students, our job isn't to call all the shots. We use a shared decision-making system within midwifery. Servant leadership is effective at both the microscale (one midwife and one client) and in a larger organizational framework (such as our midwifery college with hundreds of students and teachers). Upside-down servant leadership creates a climate where others can rise and thrive, whether that be in one family, your birth team, or a large organization.

There is real strength in this kind of servant leadership. It's not passive at all. It takes vision and courage to put others first and humility and grace to serve others well. This kind of leadership empowers, and the point of empowerment is that those we empower would take responsibility for shared goals. Whether parents or student midwives, this kind of empowerment and responsibility will invariably lead to improved outcomes in birth.

I was lucky to be mentored by quiet heroes. Because of what my early midwifery preceptors gave me, I have tried to offer that same blend of leadership and hospitality to help the hundreds of students who have passed through my life. I want them to feel the same sense of welcome and possibility that I experienced as a student. Because of what my early spiritual leaders gave me, I have tried to offer that same blend of inclusion and grace to help the thousands I have encountered in my humanitarian work. I want everyone I lead to experience that sense of belonging.

Some of us were fortunate to have mentors who modeled generous, servant-hearted leadership, while others had to find their own path without such examples. Either way, we learn from every leader we encounter and eventually decide what we want to emulate and what we refuse to repeat. With mindfulness and intention, you can choose to learn from those who lead with a spirit of nurture, encouragement, and grace. Be on the lookout for the heroes.

HISTORICAL MODELS

There are countless books and hundreds of models on leadership. Whole sections of bookstores and libraries are devoted to explaining how leaders lead, some through authority, others through charisma or influence. Unfortunately, some leaders resort to intimidation and brute force, a form of toxic leadership more akin to a dictatorship.

Throughout the ages, many leaders from different faith traditions have been profoundly influenced by studying the leadership model of Jesus and have emulated his style, bringing about significant transformation to entire nations. I think, for instance, of world leaders such as William Wilberforce in England, Reverend Dr. Martin Luther King, Jr., in the USA, and Archbishop Desmond Tutu in South Africa, all of whom credited Jesus as their inspiration. Mahatma Gandhi of India, a Hindu, said he was powerfully influenced by the teachings of Jesus, especially the Sermon on the Mount, which vividly portrays an upside-down kingdom.

"The greatest among you will be your servant," Jesus said, ushering in a new era that turned the world's model of power on its head two thousand years ago. He stands out as the leader who served, revealing that true leadership is not power over others but loving service to them. Servant leadership reveals the very heart of God, bending low to serve, lifting up the weak and weary, and leading with compassion.

STEWARDSHIP

One of the hardest things for many leaders to learn, including me, is to stop trying to control everything. Servant leadership invites a different posture: stewardship.

Stewardship means we recognize that our position is temporary, and our influence is a gift. It's not ours to hoard, it's ours to tend. We care for people and the resources we have been entrusted with, not because we own them, but because we're responsible for them.

This shift in thinking changes everything. It changes how we train others who work under us, becoming less about perfection and more about development. It changes how we handle mistakes: less about blame, more about growth. And it shifts from negative dynamics such as jealousy and competition, because stewardship prepares us to pass things on with open hands.

The longer I lead, the more I realize that holding things too tightly leads to burnout. But when we lead as stewards, we focus on building something that will last beyond us, and we can relax into that just a bit; unclench our hold and witness the breakthroughs we have been hoping and praying for.

Founders of organizations or companies sometimes hold on too tightly or for too long. However, lasting impact requires a different kind of leadership, one that is willing to let go of control, invite others into the vision, and then trust them with the dream. True leadership means serving in a way that empowers others to step into their own leadership. Watching my team carry the mission forward with strength and grace is one of the quiet rewards of servant leadership at this stage of my life.

Servant leadership naturally leads to training and equipping others. And this not only extends your impact on the world far beyond what you can do alone; it can also bring great satisfaction. I experience a special joy when I see someone that I have mentored step fully into their calling. When I witness them leading bravely and well. When I see them walk into a birth space to ease another's pain with grace and confidence. When I hear them advocating passionately for a righteous cause. When they teach skills, and I see the lightbulbs turn on for those they are instructing. And when I see them on the podium at international conferences sharing our Mercy In Action model with the world.

THE JOY OF MENTORING

A mentor has been described as a kind of guide who, despite having been far enough ahead to know something of what's down the path, comes back to walk with you. A willingness to lead involves spending time raising others. Servant leadership measures success not in personal accolades but in the growth of others. It's not about always taking the spotlight, but rather, making room for someone else to shine, and rejoicing in someone becoming empowered in their lives. I often think of the people I've had the privilege of mentoring over the years who are now out there in the world leading, and I feel so proud of what they have accomplished.

I was sitting in the back of a large conference room recently, watching as two of our midwives taught a large group of midwives and nurses from local hospitals and health centers in the Philippines. With passion and confidence, Marlene and Chesca were sharing their knowledge about our model of care, which prioritizes safety alongside respect. I knew they must have felt nervous, because the head midwife of the midwifery college that they had graduated from was in the room, but they did not let on! With conviction borne from our excellent statistics, they had the whole room leaning in as they taught on maternal and newborn survival topics. I felt such pride observing the leaders they have become!

Nerissa, another midwife I have been privileged to mentor after she lost her clinic to a natural disaster, also led an in-service that I sat in on recently. She too taught with authority, born of both experience and her hours of research, bringing updated clarity to the topics of preeclampsia and eclampsia as she deftly demonstrated the use of a newly approved IV drug and gave everyone a chance to practice. Watching leadership in action is profoundly rewarding to me.

A WELL-ROUNDED TEAM

For some of the time that I was focused on writing this book, our Mercy In Action College of Midwifery was navigating the intense reaccreditation process for our four-year bachelor of science degree. The leaders I have raised up over the years are now doing the heavy lifting in one area of our organization, so I can concentrate on another. This is remarkable, and it is only possible now because from the beginning I believed in raising others up to lead beside me. Our work has grown and thrived because I am surrounded by such a strong team of leaders, on two sides of the world. It reminds me of the well-known African proverb that my mentor, Dale Walker, used to say to me: "If you want to go fast, go alone. If you want to go far, go together."

A wise leader knows the value of surrounding themselves with people who bring different strengths to the table, and this is especially true for areas where they themselves may not excel. In other words, good leadership is not about being the best at everything, but about building a team that, together, is strong and well-rounded. Assessing both individual and team strengths and weaknesses—whether in an organization or a birth team—is one of the essential responsibilities of a leader.

A while ago I took a Leadership Orientation Instrument, which evaluates four distinct approaches to organizational leadership. The model maps scores across four categories: Structural, Political, Symbolic, and Human Resources. As I expected, I scored highest in the areas that reflect care for people and the ability to cast vision and inspire. I scored much lower in areas related to politics, negotiation, and attention to fine detail. However, when I invited seven of our senior leaders to take the same assessment and plotted all our scores on the same graph, something remarkable happened. Together, our results formed a perfect balance, with strength represented in every quadrant of the model.

RISING IN LEADERSHIP

Kristen Benoit, the director of education for our college, was still a teenager when she applied to our midwifery school in 1998. I will always remember the photo she sent with her application, grinning in a team jersey and holding a hockey stick; she looked about thirteen. But her experience told a different story. Even while balancing team sports, she was riding in the ambulance as a trained member of her small-town rescue squad and helping at the home births of her younger siblings.

After she graduated and became a licensed midwife in Vermont, Kristen and her new husband, Matt (whom she had met on the rescue squad), felt called to pursue opportunities with Mercy In Action. Just a week after the terrorist attacks on September 11, 2001, they drove across the Green Mountains to meet me at a retreat I was leading, eager to interview as full-time volunteers. In all the grief and uncertainty that week held for Americans, they offered themselves to serve wholeheartedly and without reservation.

After moving to our mission in New Mexico, Kristen began teaching midwifery beside me, while Matt did renovations on the building we would use for a mission school. They both traveled with me to Ecuador, helped lead our clinic in Mexico, and, after their first child was born, spent time living in the Philippines to establish a new birth center. When we later relocated our headquarters to Idaho, they were instrumental in launching the inaugural year of that chapter of our midwifery school, before returning to New England to continue serving from a distance while raising their family.

Quietly and without fanfare, Kristen rose through the ranks of our organization by serving, becoming so integral to our mission that she was eventually entrusted with the top leadership role in our college of midwifery. Steady and dependable, she leads as director of education from a deep well of passion and experience, continually strengthened by her pursuit of advanced education, including graduate degrees in leadership. Kristen embodies the heart of a servant leader, shaped by humility and driven by a commitment to lifelong learning. These qualities make her an invaluable presence at the helm of our college.

Matt Benoit has remained just as involved throughout the years, serving first as a volunteer builder and mechanic, and later as a primary healthcare instructor on our staff. Like Kristen, he has continued to pursue higher education while serving Mercy In Action in both volunteer and paid capacities. Today, with the experience he gained from earning a master of science in nursing leadership and management, as well as years spent leading hospital departments, Matt serves as our finance and technology director and teaches in the college.

Apart from the Penwell family, no other family has contributed as deeply or as consistently to Mercy In Action as the Benoits. They continue to add value to Mercy In Action, spending time in the Philippines each winter helping wherever and whenever it is needed. Their leadership is evident not only in the myriad ways they continue to show up with enthusiasm, but also in how they have brought members of their extended family along to champion and support our mission.

SHARED LEGACY

The leadership qualities of our staff often shine through in the way they involve their entire families in supporting our mission. Over the years, family participation of team members has been key: my parents donating an ambulance, another parent replacing damaged roofs; our sisters not only donating but managing fundraisers and offering their bookkeeping skills; siblings and cousins and nieces donating time and money; mothers, grandmothers, aunties, and kids faithfully knitting and sewing for our babies. Because they believe in the mission, everyone associated with our mission leads by sharing about it, and as a result, Mercy In Action is blessed to receive pledges and donations coming from across the generations—grandparents writing checks and grandkids donating on their smartphones! Some of our kids have shown budding leadership traits as well, rallying friends to join their knitting or sewing projects for the babies we serve, or challenging their siblings to see who can knit the most baby hats on road trips.

A unique blessing to me is how many of my past birth clients from Alaska continue to donate both financially and with goods, and their grown children do as well. A woman I midwifed for in Fairbanks more than forty years ago now knits a steady stream of hats for our Philippine babies alongside her daughter. Another couple I helped during their baby's birth in the 1980s now visit me regularly in the Philippines, as does their grown son and his wife. A few of my other "Alaska babies" have attended our schools or come to the Philippines to intern or volunteer in some way.

Over time I began to see that leadership in this work was never just about attending births. It was about welcoming families into something larger than themselves. Many of those families have continued in relationship, joining our bigger mission that reaches far beyond the day their baby was born. Generations who were touched by a single birth long ago are now impacting nations alongside us. That is the often-unseen power of legacy, one birth continuing to shape the world for generations.

SOLVING CHALLENGES CREATIVELY

We have talked about servant leadership, teamwork, and reproducing leaders. Another essential part of leadership in the midwifery sphere is creativity.

It takes creativity to serve with impact. That might sound surprising, especially if you've been taught that service is mostly about sacrifice or duty. But those of us who have spent years showing up in the broken places where systems collapse, resources are scarce, and the needs never let up, know that the most transformative service often begins with a holy imagination. We must dare to envision something better, then tap into our innate creative instincts to help bring it about.

Creative leadership in this sense isn't about talent in the arts; it's about the courage to see beyond what is and lean into what could be. It's noticing when a routine is no longer serving, when a policy is causing harm, or when someone is falling through the cracks. It's having the boldness to ask, "What if there's a better way?" and the faith to seek that better way.

Creative leadership, as I practice it, shares many commonalities with servant leadership. In both, ego takes a back seat to purpose. The goal isn't to rise to power or prove your brilliance; rather it's to lift others higher and improve the lives of those in need. And often, the most powerful way to lift others is by redesigning the very systems that have been holding them down.

That's why creative leadership matters so much in midwifery. Our work is full of adaptive challenges. Adaptive challenges are defined as the kinds of issues that can't be fixed by simply applying technical knowledge or doing what's always been done. They are problems that don't come with a clear solution or a manual to follow. Instead, adaptive challenges require us to gain new perspectives, learn something new, involve others, and sometimes rethink our assumptions entirely.

Adaptive challenges by their very nature call for creativity, humility, collaboration, and the courage to try and fail repeatedly until we figure it out. We serve real people with complex lives, working with limited resources, and in real time, without the luxury of hindsight until much later. It takes imagination to improve anything under those conditions, and sometimes it takes imagination just to make things work at all.

So press in, treat creative leadership as an act of resistance, and see what becomes possible.

DESIGN THEORY

Design theory, a component of creative leadership, teaches us that the most effective innovations often begin with deep empathy. Before we begin to solve, we must listen. Before we seek to fix, we must feel. That sounds like midwifery, doesn't it? We lean in, we observe closely, we ask questions. We need to do the same thing when we are problem-solving a leadership dilemma as when we are attending a labor.

Creative leaders often borrow the principles of design and apply them directly to our settings: What does this mother need to feel safe? What would make this clinic more welcoming? How could our team communicate more clearly in emergencies? What behaviors do we need to start building to earn more trust? What are the barriers to someone being able to be cared for by us, and how can we remove them? What's not working, and what if we tried it another way? The best ideas begin with seeing the world through someone else's eyes and caring enough to respond.

Mimee, an Indigenous woman, served as a catalyst by exposing a critical issue that prompted us to seek a solution. She and her family were living in a resettlement camp, still displaced decades after the eruption of Mount Pinatubo in the Philippines, which was one of the most powerful volcanic eruptions of the twentieth century. When the volcano erupted in 1991, it buried entire communities in ash and mud, displacing tens of thousands of Indigenous Aeta families. Even twenty years later, many were still living in makeshift housing with limited access to healthcare, clean water, and transportation. At the time we met her, Mimee was pregnant but unable to afford the fare from the resettlement camp to our birth center for prenatal care or delivery.

In another setting, we would have offered home-based care, but where I live in the Philippines, they now have an effective ban on midwives providing labor and delivery services for women in their homes. In response, we created a new policy, ensuring the entire tribal resettlement community was aware that we would cover transportation costs for all pregnant women in the camp. Word spread quickly, and after Mimee gave birth at our birth center and reported back that not only was all care free, but we had kept our word to pay the taxi fare to get her there, Aeta women began arriving in labor in the middle of the night. That one small act of empathy-based problem-solving made safer birth possible for an entire community.

Sometimes when I talk about using creativity, people say to me, "Oh, but I'm not creative like you." To that I say: Everyone is creative in their own way. Creativity is part of our human birthright, but we often keep it to ourselves or discard it as we grow from children into self-conscious adults. We were made to adapt, to build, to reimagine the world around us. Creativity begins with vision. But acting on our creative ideas requires courage and a deliberate choice, and some people do not want to take the risk.

If servant leadership gives us our posture, then creative leadership gives us our tools. We serve by imagining a better world. We lead by making room for others to imagine a better world with us. There is no limit to the solutions we can discover and bring to life together if we have a shared vision of the way we want things to be, and we don't care who gets the credit.

Midwifery that improves outcomes requires this blend of heart and ingenuity. There will always be some who cling to what's familiar, who resist change at every turn. But those of us who feel called to serve with vision and lead with hope in hard places must be willing to stretch our imaginations and welcome others into the process.

FROM OBSERVATION TO INNOVATION

Creative leadership often begins with simply paying attention. In our birth work, we're trained to observe. We notice tone and tension, as well as subtle shifts in behavior or breathing. We're wired to scan for patterns and pick up on what's missing. These same instincts for practiced attentiveness are the soil where creative leadership takes root.

Every innovation, at its core, starts with noticing a problem. When something feels clunky or inefficient, when a mother leaves a visit feeling confused, or when a student midwife is struggling to master a skill but is afraid to speak up, these are all invitations into creative leadership. They are small doors into the bigger question: Is this an opportunity to do what we do better?

Tom and David Kelley, in their book *Creative Confidence*, remind us that the most powerful innovations often come not from technical genius but from empathy. As leaders, this way of thinking gives us a pathway. It teaches us to observe and empathize, define the problem, imagine new solutions, and then test and refine them until they work. Studying creative leadership as a concept helped me do what I was already doing in midwifery, but with greater intention and a sharper focus on impact.

The kind of leadership we need in birth culture today is not defined by titles or rigid roles. It is marked by responsiveness, vision, and the willingness to change when change is needed. We need leaders who keep both eyes open, who notice the gaps, and who care enough to step into them. We need leaders who are not afraid to let go of outdated methods when they no longer serve the people in our care.

Leadership rooted in empathy and courage, shaped by careful observation, and followed by meaningful action is what gives rise to true innovation. And when that innovation is guided by love and grounded in humility, it has the power to improve lives and reshape outcomes, which is something that can be measured over time through birth statistics.

NOBODY SAID IT WAS EASY

M. Scott Peck starts his book *The Road Less Traveled* with the stark declaration, "Life is difficult." We could also say, "Leadership is difficult." It is not glamorous, and most of us don't seek it out for its own sake. We lead because we've seen what happens when systems are broken, when care is disrespectful and unsafe, and when no one cares enough or dares to think differently and try something new.

Leadership of the kind that impacts birth outcomes is rarely easy. I have heard it said that most people reject being leaders because they want to have an easy life, but I don't think that is true for midwives, because we already chose a hard life! So let's make it count by being willing to lead when the need arises. Remember, you don't need to wear the title "leader" to lead. You only need the courage to act on what you know is right and the imagination to see what could be possible if we are willing to serve and bring others along with us on the journey.

Because I never set out to be a leader, in my early years of midwifery I tried at every opportunity to give it away to someone I thought was more qualified. I kept saying that I just wanted to serve, not be the leader. But over time, as I said yes to more leadership needs because no one else was there to do it, I discovered something important: Leadership, when rooted in humility, becomes one of the highest forms of service.

There's often a redemptive arc in a leader's life if you look closely. The Filipina midwives I work with have all known suffering. Everyone on our American leadership team has faced unique challenges and heartbreak. One of the clearest markers of authentic leadership is the ability to walk through adversity, unwanted change, or crisis and come out not just surviving, but stronger. The very skills that help someone face hardship and come through more committed than ever are the same ones that shape great leaders.

All leaders have moments of victory and moments of failure; times of feeling exhilaration and times of struggle. Expect both. I don't know of a single leader who has never felt discouraged, but the great ones don't give up the fight. Because the alternative to leadership is standing on the sidelines when something important is happening and choosing to do nothing. For me, that would be harder. Which *hard* would you rather do?

In his 1910 speech *Citizenship in a Republic*, Theodore Roosevelt spoke words that still resonate today:

> It is not the critic who counts; not the man who points out how the strong man stumbles, or where the doer of deeds could have done them better. The credit belongs to the man who is actually in the arena, whose face is marred by dust and sweat and blood; who strives valiantly; who errs, who comes short again and again, because there is no effort without error and shortcoming; but who does actually strive to do the deeds; who knows the great enthusiasms, the great devotions; who spends himself in a worthy cause; who at the best knows in the end the triumph of high achievement, and who at the worst, if he fails, at least fails while daring greatly, so that his place shall never be with those cold and timid souls who neither know victory nor defeat.

Leadership is not for the faint of heart, and if you are doing a good job of supporting the people you lead, expect to take a few hits. It has been said that the tall trees catch the hurricane winds. Another similar saying I've often heard is that if you stick your head up out of the trenches, someone will shoot at it. Expect that. Those hits are not a sign that you're doing something wrong—they're often evidence that you're standing for something that matters.

I once heard a story:

A man died and approached St. Peter at the pearly gates.

"What does it take to get in?" he asked.

"Show me your scars," St. Peter said.

"I don't have any."

St. Peter paused. "How sad. Was there nothing down there worth fighting for?"

SLEEVES ROLLED UP

Midwifery as it should be is a picture of servant leadership with its sleeves rolled up: a strong team working together to serve each individual mother, baby, and family unit. It's leading because love compels us.

Servant leadership doesn't mean we lose ourselves, but it does mean serving and mentoring even when our own reserves feel low, and maybe at times without thanks. It means we lead from our truest self. From the part of us that's rooted in purpose, not ego. From the part that still remembers why we said yes to this work in the first place.

The best leaders I know are not trying to be impressive or gain a name for themselves. They're trying to be useful. They want to make the world a better place. They don't lead from ego, but from a deep connection to their purpose. That's what I hope this chapter stirs in you. Not pressure to lead like someone else, but the courage to lead as yourself. To lead with vision, because you can see what needs to be done. To lead with confidence even when it feels unfamiliar or uncomfortable, simply because there are people to serve, and you are willing and able to do so with excellence.

LEADING TOWARD EXCELLENCE

Excellence is never an accident; it is always the result of intention, effort, and a conscious choice to do things right. This is true in both clinical and academic settings. It takes a visionary leader to ensure excellence is achieved, one who can appreciate why good leadership is key to growing future leaders and improving birth outcomes. However excellent a leader is, they can exponentially multiply their impact by nurturing other leaders and releasing them to spread their wings.

HOPE FOR THE FUTURE

Every movement for meaningful change depends on strong, dynamic leadership. We must have hope for the future to lead well, because a good leader needs to help people overcome cynicism. Having glimpsed the hearts and minds of hundreds of students and midwives as I teach workshops around the world, I retain a deep and abiding hope in the emerging generation of leaders who are out there waiting to be inspired to action.

In Part Two we will explore creativity in birth work and describe some strategies for how to move from vision to action. I'll share some of the practical innovations my team and I have envisioned and implemented, along with a few helpful frameworks we've adopted and adapted over the years. These creative practices have played a significant role in some of our most meaningful successes in the birth world, and I'm excited to share them with you, in the hope they may prove useful in your own settings.

PAUSE FOR REFLECTION

Have you ever sensed a calling to lead, yet found yourself hesitating to fully step into that role? When you reflect on the leaders you've encountered in birth work, have they modeled nurturing servant leadership or self-serving leadership? How could you use your influence to mentor someone else?

PART II

A CULTURE OF SERVING WITH CREATIVITY

INNOVATIONS AND ADAPTATIONS

A Tale of Labor and Birth: Evangeline's Story

This story is based on the experience of a woman who delivered her baby in our birth center in an impoverished community in the Philippines, where dwellings cluster around a slaughterhouse and the local cemetery is home to a squatter population.

Clutching the arm of her husband, Evangeline walks around a corner and onto a narrow side street. At almost midnight in this neighborhood called Lorega, the streets are awash with flickering lights, candles, small fires burning, and the occasional bare light bulb, hanging from a cord draped over makeshift poles and running on borrowed electricity. Wrapping around her like a heavy blanket, the humid air carries the mingled scents of frying fish, kerosene smoke, and open drains. The sound of dogs barking in the distance echoes between the shanties, blending with the laughter of children and the murmur of voices that fill every corner of the night.

Even at this late hour, groups of children run and play, chasing each other in and out of alleyways. Men squat beside the narrow street, their backs against the two-story wooden shacks that line the path, cigarettes gleaming with red embers at each inhale. Mothers with babies in their arms or on their backs talk and laugh with each other, occasionally stopping to grab an errant child out of harm's way. From their upstairs windows, old grannies watch the night in silence, missing nothing.

Past the slaughterhouse, stepping over rivulets of blood that run down the street, Evangeline walks slowly, for it is a heavy burden she carries. The squealing of pigs rends the night air, animal sounds of terror, but no one pays any attention; it is the every-night sound. The metallic smell of blood from the slaughterhouse clings to her nostrils, and she feels her stomach turn, yet she presses forward, gripping tighter her husband's arm.

Alongside the cemetery where the living share space with the dead, they walk slowly, skirting around makeshift memorials. Evangeline shudders as she passes the shadowy tombs, not knowing yet what the night will hold for her. She understands, at least in part, the role she is about to assume tonight and senses the gravity of the hour before her, accepting both the peril and the promise it may hold.

Down a slight incline and around to the left she advances with her beloved, past the sari-sari stores with their meager displays of candies, soda bottles, and soaps all hung in strips dangling from the ceiling. A radio plays somewhere nearby, its tinny speaker offering a '70s love song that drifts through the night air. Steam rises from the food stalls, curling upward and catching the glow of the lights, making halos in the smoke as they pass the pots of rice and pansit noodles for sale. Past the crowds of men who gamble in the streets and past the drug pushers, she slowly navigates her way, never letting go of the strong arm at her side. She notices everything and she notices nothing, for tonight her senses are focused on this strange new sensation, a rhythmic pulling and dragging down low in her belly. At times, the pain causes her to gasp and catch her breath, and then she continues on down the street.

Evangeline sees her destination now as she rounds the last corner: a square two-story building surrounded by a green cement fence. The lights are burning brightly here, and sounds of activity float out the windows into the night air: a baby's cry, a laugh, the happy sounds of people who work and live together and like each other. The building seems almost to glow, a beacon of order and safety in a sea of chaos, and her heart lifts at the sight. She comes to the gate and rings the bell. In the moonlight, she can read the words painted in white: Mercy In Action Free Maternity Clinic.

The door opens, and kind hands reach for her, smiles and exclamations usher her in: "Tonight's your night! Welcome, welcome!" The smell of clean linens and freshly scrubbed floors greets her, comforting in its promise of care. Inside, soft voices blend with the low hum of a fan, and she feels the tension begin to leave her shoulders. A little while later, examined and reassured that all is well, she is ensconced in a small but tidy room. White sheets dress the bed, and lace curtains billow from the window. A large oxygen tank stands sentinel in the corner, as medical supplies perch inside a carved wooden dresser with glass-front doors.

Evangeline relaxes into the rhythm of the night, into the rhythm of pain. One midwife stays with her now, never sleeping, keeping a constant watch, praying, nurturing, loving. Each time the midwife presses the Doppler to her belly, the baby's heart answers at once, a fast, reassuring beat-beat-beat that drums through the room and gives Evangeline hope.

As her labor nears transition, a second midwife enters the room quietly, and each time they touch her arm or offer water to her lips, she feels strength to continue, their gentle presence a balm to her fleeting thoughts of fear.

Come the dawn, weary but oh-so grateful, Evangeline will open her arms to receive a perfect little miracle. As the first rays of sunlight spill through the window, gilding her newborn's face, she will look over and smile at her astonished husband, and for one small moment, the world itself will seem to pause, as life begins anew in Lorega.

5
MISSION-DRIVEN MODELS AND FRAMEWORKS

There is no power for change greater than a community discovering what it cares about.

— MARGARET WHEATLEY

IN MY DECADES OF WORKING ALONGSIDE MIDWIVES IN MANY COUNTRIES, I have seen firsthand how midwifery care changes outcomes for entire communities. I think of the pregnant women who arrive at our birth centers in the Philippines after being turned away from hospitals because they had no money. In those moments, when they are welcomed in the door in advanced labor, our open access model has been a lifeline, restoring safety and respect to families who had been denied both.

What makes good care possible is more than the presence of skilled midwives; it is the presence of the models and frameworks that guide us and hold us accountable. The International Childbirth Initiative and the Safe Motherhood Initiative remind us that maternity care must be accessible, evidence-based, and respectful. The midwifery model of care reminds us of our scope of practice, values, and duty.

The open access model reminds us of our compassion and humanity, and the three-delays model reminds us of the dangers of not paying attention or not having a plan. Midwives working within these frameworks meet families where they are, providing care without discrimination, and upholding the truth that every mother, baby, and family deserves to survive and to thrive with dignity during pregnancy, childbirth, and after.

THE MIDWIFERY MODEL

Midwives comprise the largest group of maternity care providers globally. The World Health Organization (WHO) and the International Confederation of Midwives (ICM) promote and define the implementation of midwifery models of care as a universal approach. The midwifery model of care is trademarked as the Midwives Model of Care in America. It is a system of maternity care built on respect and informed consent. Midwives working within this model specialize in supporting the normal, physiological process of birth, offering woman-centered, personalized care and shared decision-making.

Though experts in normal birth, midwives in this model are also trained in essential emergency skills, prepared to act swiftly when complications arise. The midwifery model's unique blend of respect for the natural process of human reproduction and the skilled use of lifesaving measures when needed is what leads to the superior outcomes and patient satisfaction that Mercy in Action has recorded for decades.

However, the midwifery model of care, while practiced by many midwives worldwide, is not exclusive to midwives nor inherently tied to the title itself. Some physicians are deeply committed to protecting and supporting women's wishes for a natural birth and are extremely kind and respectful during the process of labor. My colleague André LaLonde, an obstetrician who has acted as a consultant to WHO, reminded me while I was writing this chapter that there are birthing facilities that, while not midwife-led, do practice family-centered maternity care, a philosophy that prioritizes safe and respectful maternity practices and centers the needs of the mother and baby.

On the other hand, I have been in many settings where midwives are trained in overly medicalized approaches and were unkind and even abusive during a delivery. And I have seen places where midwives were not allowed to learn emergency skills or even basic suturing, because they were considered just lowly assistants to the doctors within a hierarchical system.

For the midwifery model of care to flourish, it must be practiced within systems that allow its full expression. Reimagining birth culture means creating environments where midwifery is honored and supported, for the sake of mothers and babies. This is best accomplished using models and frameworks available that are tested and proven to work.

REAL DANGER

The danger faced by women giving birth is real. In the nearly five decades I have been practicing as a midwife, progress has been made in reducing the maternal and infant mortality rates, yet today a mother still dies every two minutes from pregnancy and childbirth-related causes somewhere in the world. Mortality rates vary greatly by country, but the staggering truth is that the vast majority of this burden of death falls on the poorest countries, about equally divided between Asia and Africa. This is not only a health crisis, but also a matter of deep injustice within our global family.

When I first began working in Southeast Asia in 1990, no one was talking about the things I was witnessing. I saw shocking physical and emotional abuse in hospitals at the hands of doctors, nurses, and midwives who should have been helping, not harming, mothers and babies during labor and birth.

Today, abuse and disrespect in childbirth are still a problem, but it is no longer hidden. The world is talking about it, and the pressure is on for respectful maternity care to become the standard everywhere. Abuse and disrespect in childbirth, called obstetric violence by some, is now documented and discussed in diverse circles. From the White Ribbon Alliance to Amnesty International, from Harvard University to the pages of the *International Journal of Gynecology & Obstetrics* and *Midwifery Today* magazine, practitioners, researchers, and the public are calling for change. This is an encouraging and vitally important shift, because acknowledging and documenting a problem is the first step to solving it. However, it is only the first step.

Although women's groups and human rights advocates around the globe are calling for respect in childbirth, the focus of many health professionals, policymakers, and lawmakers is often solely on improving physical safety. At times, these goals of safety and respect appear to be in conflict, which they should never be. I always remember my Dutch midwife friend Beatrijs Smulders telling me when I attended a home birth with her in Amsterdam early in my career that a good birth *is* a safe birth. And I believe the reverse is true also; a safe birth should be experienced by the mother as a good birth.

It is appropriate that individual healthcare professionals, alongside governments, NGOs, and mission agencies, are working around the world to improve survival rates surrounding childbirth. Increasingly, the conversation has gone deeper, recognizing that policies around childbirth practices must never deny human rights.

As someone who has witnessed abusive behaviors in delivery rooms firsthand in Southeast Asia, Latin America, and even parts of the United States, I know I am not alone in longing for a different reality. My heart hurts especially for the poor and marginalized who suffer most from a lack of safety and respect in childbirth. If we want better outcomes, how we treat pregnant women has to become a matter of life and death.

Still, long-standing patterns of behavior that harm women are not easily ended, particularly in cultures where women have few rights to begin with. Rules, policies, and cultural norms alike can violate the fundamental human rights of mothers, babies, and families during the vulnerable time of pregnancy and childbirth. Yet it has been proven that these human rights violations do not lead to safer deliveries; abuse, neglect, and non-consensual care just make birth more dangerous.

Knowing that excessive medicalization can be just as dangerous, both physically and emotionally, as neglect and undertreatment, we need a clear path to the Goldilocks zone, where care is just right. Fortunately, there are researchers and authors who stand beside the midwifery community with visionary minds and compassionate hearts, dedicating their careers to studying the problems and guiding us toward solutions. Suellen Miller, Melissa Cheyney, and Robbie Davis-Floyd are three such women. They have all researched and written extensively on the extremes of excessive medicalization and extreme neglect in maternity care, working individually and together to shape a new way of seeing an old problem. In the process, they have helped shape my own thinking about how to develop strategies that carefully avoid the pitfalls of poor choices made by either "too much too soon" or "too little too late" when it comes to interventions in childbirth.

TOO MUCH TOO SOON AND TOO LITTLE TOO LATE

A conceptual framework has been created to address the reality that childbirth care often falls into two dangerous extremes. In a landmark *Lancet* article coauthored by midwife Suellen Miller, these were described as "too little, too late" (TLTL) and "too much, too soon" (TMTS). TLTL refers to care that is given with inadequate resources, below evidence-based standards, or withheld due to lack of ability to pay for services or discrimination. This failure is a driving force behind high maternal and newborn mortality and morbidity, especially in low-resource settings where women and babies often face difficulty accessing care in time.

One example of TLTL is the underutilization of cesarean births, when there is no one trained to assist, or no functional operating theater, or when there is simply no access to a medical facility when a woman or a baby is in danger. A cesarean delivery is generally needed for birth around 10% of the time, yet in some parts of rural Africa and Asia, rates are less than half that.

On the opposite side is TMTS, the routine over-medicalization of normal pregnancy and birth. This includes the unnecessary use of potentially harmful procedures without supporting evidence, as well as the overuse of interventions that can save lives when needed but become harmful when applied indiscriminately. To use the example of cesareans again, overuse of surgery for birth represents this extreme, with cesarean rates double what is recommended globally and as high as 90% in some private hospitals. While the cesarean has become a relatively safe operation, any surgery carries risk. Cesarean sections are associated with a roughly threefold higher risk of maternal mortality compared to vaginal deliveries and carry higher risks of severe bleeding, infection, and venous thromboembolism.

Strategic midwifery seeks to navigate wisely between these two extremes, protecting normal physiological birth while ensuring that skilled, lifesaving interventions are available when truly needed. Suellen, who also coauthored the popular Hesperian Foundation's *A Book for Midwives* and helped develop clinical trials for the non-pneumatic anti-shock garment (NASG), epitomizes this. Her work shows that both prevention and emergency response are equally needed to save lives during childbirth.

My friend Robbie is a brilliant medical anthropologist who has spent her life researching and writing about birth models around the world. Robbie has written and lectured on exemplary models, as well as identifying systems that are failing to serve the people they are meant to help. I was humbled and honored when she asked me to write a chapter on Mercy In Action that was published in her 2009 book, *Birth Models That Work*.

According to Robbie's research, effective birth models are maternity care systems that excel in several key ways, including supporting and enabling normal physiological birth by minimizing unnecessary or non-evidence-based interventions. At the same time, the care system should be fully capable of responding to complications when birth veers from normal, offering skilled and appropriate care when it is most needed. In order to be included in her definition of a birth model that works, the model must consistently deliver excellent outcomes, not only in terms of maternal and newborn health but also in terms of emotional and psychological satisfaction for mothers and families.

To have Mercy In Action recognized as a living example of this philosophy in practice was a great validation of our visionary midwifery model. Our birth centers in the Philippines have consistently shown that it is possible to achieve excellent outcomes among a mixed-risk population living below the poverty line, while treating families with utmost dignity and respect.

RIGHT AMOUNT, RIGHT TIME, RIGHT WAY

Robbie, together with her fellow PhD anthropologist Melissa Cheyney, a midwife, coauthored an article suggesting a reframing of the dichotomy of too little too late or too much too soon. In response to the polar-opposite problems of TLTL and TMTS in childbirth, they proposed a commonsense phrase: care that is "the right amount at the right time in the right way," abbreviated as RARTRW. Shouldn't everyone receive healthcare that is "just right"?

One of the greatest challenges in achieving this optimal maternity care has been the absence of a shared framework, a clear set of standards to measure whether the care given during childbirth is truly in the best interests of the mother, baby, and the entire family. Most facilities where babies are born act in isolation, with little to no collaboration with other facilities. In these places, problems tend to persist on both ends of the spectrum: Maternity care that is "too little, too late" continues to threaten lives, while a "too much too soon" management style of attempting to control labor and birth has become increasingly recognized as dangerous. When everyone is working from a vastly different playbook, it is the recipients of care who suffer.

INTERNATIONAL CHILDBIRTH INITIATIVE

This is where the International Childbirth Initiative comes in, offering us all a common, evidence-based framework. Its "12 steps to safe and respectful MotherBaby-Family maternity care" are clear, practical, and measurable, and they carry the weight of international consensus. Directing us to evidence-based care, and emphasizing respect throughout, the steps unite us around the shared goals of improving outcomes for every mother giving birth in any setting. When birth is protected in this way, we can save lives and protect human rights, honoring the whole person, body, soul, and spirit.

The International Childbirth Initiative (ICI): 12 Steps to Safe and Respectful MotherBaby-Family Maternity Care provides a clear path for making positive changes in the way childbirth is approached. One strength of the initiative lies in its universality, as it is not written for any one profession, but rather for birthing facilities where midwives, obstetricians, pediatricians, doulas, and nurses can agree on principles and behaviors that their own international organizations have already endorsed.

Another strength of the ICI lies in its scope: twelve steps that carry far more weight than anything a single practitioner or facility could accomplish alone. Internationally, it holds unique credibility, as it was not developed by a single nation or group, but rather through a survey of medical and women's organizations and the collaboration of experts worldwide.

Once after I had shared about our birth center at a local health department meeting, the doctor serving as health director of our barangay in the Philippines came up to me with a frown and said, "I do not think I am comfortable with you not performing episiotomy on first-time mothers." For a split second I was speechless and my mind searched for an answer. Then I said, "Actually, step seven in the International Childbirth Initiative recommends that we perform episiotomy only when it is medically indicated for a specific complication, not as a routine procedure. Could I show you the evidence for that step?"

It turned out to be the perfect response to defuse the tension. Later that week I followed up and shared the ICI document with him. Surprisingly, the following month at the health department meeting, that same doctor came up to me again, this time with a wide smile. "We have also stopped routinely giving episiotomies to every woman," he said. "I just wanted you to know we want to be evidence-based, too."

This is an example of how using a framework based on evidence can be a perfect strategy for bridging differences in approach. Using the ICI gave me a framework that carried authority beyond my own opinion, and it opened the door for constructive dialogue. I find that being a part of this larger initiative changes the unhelpful narratives around birth that tend to pit doctors against midwives, or one country's style of doing things against another country's way of doing that same thing. ICI is bigger, does not belong to any one country, and has documented credible resources to support each step. It is not a battle of ideologies around birth care but rather a common set of steps that a birth facility has agreed to uphold, and by which every practice decision can be measured.

The ICI offers a roadmap for providing care that is the right amount, at the right time, in the right way (RARTRW). The International

Childbirth Initiative serves as a framework in hundreds of hospitals, birth centers, and home birth settings in dozens of countries, and has been translated into more than twenty languages so far. It helps remind us all about this balance as we provide care and create policy.

ICI STEPS

In a nutshell, Step 1 establishes the foundation of respectful care. Step 2 calls for maternity care that is accessible, affordable, and nondiscriminatory. The focus of Steps 3 through 8 is on keeping childbirth normal. Specifically, Step 3 calls for care that is evidence-based, values-driven, and responsive to the needs of women, babies, and families. Step 4 asserts that every woman has the right to continuous support in labor and birth. Step 5 encourages the use of non-pharmaceutical comfort measures, with full information provided when medications are considered. Step 6 promotes specific evidence-based practices throughout pregnancy, birth, and postpartum. Step 7 names and cautions against routine or harmful interventions that lack evidence of benefit. Step 8 emphasizes prevention and wellness through the lens of social determinants of health such as nutrition, hygiene, family planning, and health education.

With Step 9, the focus shifts to ensuring that when birth complications arise, skilled emergency care is available and delivered with excellence. Steps 10 and 11 emphasize teamwork and good working conditions to optimize outcomes regardless of the course labor takes. Finally, Step 12 incorporates the 10 Steps of the Baby-Friendly Hospital Initiative put together by the WHO and UNICEF, reinforcing best practices in breastfeeding support.

ACCOUNTABILITY

Each step is measurable and grounded in accountability, with progress tracked through questionnaires that a woman completes after giving birth. There is also a survey for the family members who witnessed the treatment she received; both the women's and the family questionnaire are directly tied to the 12 steps and how well they were followed during her birth experience in the facility.

To ensure the responses are accurate in our birth centers, we have hired a cultural liaison to oversee our surveys and speak directly with patients after they complete their discharge questionnaires if they have any questions or concerns. Rina Miller is a Filipina, fluent in three languages, and is not a care provider herself. She also gave birth three times in two different Mercy In Action sponsored birth centers, making her ideal for the role. Our midwives use the feedback from these surveys and interviews to identify ways to improve our care.

NO FALSE CHOICES

The ICI speaks directly to a question I have heard many times from well-intentioned providers of maternity care: "Which is more important? Safety for mother and baby, or a gentle, respectful birth experience for the mother?" The ICI 12 steps don't force us to choose, and that is one of the things I love most about this framework. Half of the steps focus on protecting the natural processes of birth and breastfeeding, while the other half concentrate on safeguarding mothers and babies through prevention and treatment of complications that may arise. The balance is striking, and the guidance is entirely practical, helping providers honor both safety and respect in every situation.

Importantly, the steps put the needs of the family having a baby at the center, where they belong. In fact, the ICI has a distinctive approach to speaking about the family, and this is another way they avoid a fool's choice. They intentionally join the words *mother*, *baby*, and *family* without spaces between the words *mother* and *baby*. I often have to explain that MotherBaby-Family is not a typo, but a statement of both reality and values. Mother and baby are always represented in ICI documents as one word because they are one unit, a dyad whose mutual well-being is inseparable.

This truth begins in pregnancy, where everything that affects the mother inevitably affects the baby, and it continues after birth through the first hours, days, and weeks. The ICI Initiative reminds us that the care of mothers and babies should never be separated, either in practice or in policy. Early skin-to-skin contact, initiation of breastfeeding, and keeping mothers and babies together are not luxuries but essentials, because the health of one depends on the other.

The addition of the word *family* completes the picture, acknowledging that mother and baby belong within a wider circle of love and support. By holding the MotherBaby-Family together in this way, the ICI framework calls us to honor the deep bonds of connection and to shape maternity care that safeguards not only survival but also relationship, attachment, and belonging. The initiative reminds us that pregnancy, birth, postpartum, and early infancy unfold within a larger circle of community, even in the most complex situations.

ICI cuts to the heart of strategic midwifery and is a model for safety and respect in childbirth that works in every setting, everywhere in the world. Any facility where babies are born, from a large teaching hospital to a small independent birth center, can become an implementing partner of the International Childbirth Initiative.

Mercy In Action uses the International Childbirth Initiative as a guiding framework in every setting where we serve. Whether we are introducing ourselves to a new community, training midwives and doctors, or responding in the midst of disaster, the ICI 12 Steps have provided us with both credibility and direction. We have taught them in hospitals and birth centers, woven them into online courses and seminars, and carried them into makeshift birth tents. They have shaped our capacity-building programs, anchored our cultural competency training, and served as the framework I point to when consulting with others. Again and again, the ICI has proven to be a birth model that works anywhere, and we find that following the steps consistently leads to better outcomes for mothers, babies, and entire families.

The International Childbirth Initiative (ICI), along with its predecessors the International MotherBaby Childbirth Initiative and the Mother-Friendly and Baby-Friendly initiatives, has provided a framework that Mercy In Action has relied on since the early 1990s. This framework has evolved and stood the test of time. In fact, Mercy In Action values the principles embodied by these steps so much that we only financially support birth centers that are committed to formally implementing all 12 steps of the ICI.

PACKING FOR DISASTER

As we packed for the journey into the heart of the disaster zone left behind after the largest storm on Earth tore through the islands to our south, every item had to count. I knew our space was limited to what we could fit in our ambulance and the backpacks strapped to each of our team members. Anything we brought had to be essential, and anything we forgot could cost lives. The hospitals were smashed, the clinics flattened, and people were in desperate need of care.

As I scanned our supply list one more time, I told our team to remember to bring the binder with the Steps, knowing that in the chaos to come, when care would be offered by many hands and countless volunteers, we would need a compass to guide us. That binder was more than just words on paper. Following a framework like the 12 Steps of ICI is a constant reminder that even in disaster, when there are many potential excuses to cut corners, we are still called to the highest standards of safe and respectful care.

When I shared about our experiences after returning from the disaster zone, one of the founding members of the International Childbirth Initiative remarked that if Mercy In Action could uphold all the Steps in a makeshift disaster tent with no electricity, scarce resources, and patients who were homeless and traumatized, with even food and clean water in short supply, then anyone could do it!

THREE DELAYS FRAMEWORK

A different kind of framework we use to keep our care top-notch is the Three Delays, a well-known concept in global maternal health. This framework helps anyone attending a labor to identify the most common points where the mother or baby may be at risk. I often call it the Three Deadly Delays, because the delays are known to lead to higher rates of maternal, fetal, and newborn death.

Here is what to be aware of and avoid: (1) delay in recognizing a problem and deciding to seek care, (2) delay in starting emergency treatment outside a hospital and/or reaching a facility, and (3) delay in receiving appropriate care once the patient arrives at a hospital or higher-level facility.

Understanding the concept of the three delays is crucial. The first deadly delay is the time it takes to recognize that something is wrong. This can happen during pregnancy, labor, or the postpartum period, a time when we know many maternal deaths occur. But mostly we look at delays in recognizing a problem in labor. The question is, how long does it take before someone realizes there is a problem?

Delays at this stage may happen for a multitude of reasons. Sometimes vital signs are not assessed often enough (or at all) to detect early warning signs, due to a provider's carelessness, busyness, or not wanting to disturb the mother. Some births have no skilled birth attendant present to measure the blood pressure, pulse, respirations, and temperature.

Hypertension, fetal distress, or shock initially go undetected without careful monitoring, until it is too late. At other times, the signs of a medical complication may be present but not recognized due to gaps in training, a lack of respect for warning signs, or even denial. Exhaustion can also play a role, clouding judgment and slowing reaction time. Personal attachment may be a factor as well. Midwives know how to watch for the red flags, but have admitted after an adverse outcome that the affection they feel and the desire to support a mother's birth plan can lead to overlooking the accumulation of small pink flags.

The second deadly delay is the time it takes to respond to the problem or to reach a higher level of care. I break this delay into two parts. First, how long does it take the attendant present at the birth to respond when they do recognize a clear abnormality? And second, if transfer becomes necessary, how long does it take to reach a hospital or a higher-level or tertiary care hospital?

Often, discussions of the three delays picture a rural woman without a trained attendant, relying on relatives to put her on a makeshift stretcher and carry her to the distant hospital. That is one reality. However, in many out-of-hospital settings, the key question is how quickly the birth professional attending the birth can initiate emergency care while urgently arranging transport to higher-level care. Or, in some cases, if the birth attendant acts quickly, a hospital transfer may not be necessary at all, because the problem was resolved before harm was done.

Why does the second delay happen? Perhaps the required medication is not readily available, or restrictive laws prevent midwives from administering the emergency drug. Perhaps the emergency equipment is hard to access, such as when IV supplies are scattered throughout the birth bag instead of being consolidated and easily accessible at a moment's notice. Perhaps the oxygen is cold from being left in the car in winter and must be warmed before administering to someone in shock. And remember the problem of vehicles mentioned earlier? Transport issues can cause a delay even in developed countries if the transport vehicle's gas tank is not kept full or tires and engines are not maintained.

The third deadly delay is the time it takes to receive treatment once the woman arrives at a referral hospital. There is often a sense of relief during a transport upon reaching a medical facility, but delays can still occur at that stage, a phenomenon I have witnessed not only in resource-limited settings but also in hospitals in America. The delays in the hospital initiating treatment may be caused by shortages of skilled personnel, lack of essential equipment or supplies, poor management, or inadequate emergency obstetric care protocols. It could also be due to conscious or unconscious bias against home birth.

The solutions to the three delays are both practical and strategic. Timely, consistent monitoring of vitals must be non-negotiable. Safeguards must be built into midwifery practice to minimize fatigue and denial, including working in pairs so one midwife is always rested enough to make good decisions. Assigning roles at every birth—one midwife for the baby, one for the mother—prevents critical details from being overlooked in the event of simultaneous complications. We may need to advocate for new laws around access to lifesaving drugs at out of hospital births. We must build relationships with staff at referral hospitals and reach agreements before a transfer is needed.

These delays are called deadly for a reason: They cost lives. Strategic midwifery means recognizing where the risks lie and putting systems in place to prevent or mitigate harm before it causes bad outcomes in childbirth.

At Mercy In Action, we use this three-delays model as another lens to help us see clearly what we need to do for the best outcome. This grounds us in what is actually happening at a labor, rather than what we wish was happening or thought would happen. It helps us address the social, cultural, and systemic barriers that can lead to tragedy if birth becomes complicated. By working to reduce each of these delays through education, accessibility, timely transport, adequate supply stock, and skilled, respectful care, we position midwives to save lives in any setting.

The three delays explain why mothers and babies are still dying, and the ICI provides evidence-based, respectful solutions that address those gaps, ensuring that families can receive the quality of care and the compassion they deserve. Next, let's look at a tool for avoiding some of the delays while following the ICI's 12 steps.

BIRTH PREPAREDNESS AND COMPLICATION READINESS FRAMEWORK

If you have a car sitting in your driveway, even an old one that barely runs, you have more wealth than the majority of people in the world. When working in low-resource areas, one reason we need to plan ahead for when labor begins is that approximately 80% of people worldwide do not own a vehicle. This is where the Birth Preparedness and Complication Readiness framework is a game changer for those of us living in low-resource, high-mortality countries like the Philippines.

LOW-RESOURCE COUNTRY PLAN

In 2006, we moved to a remote island community where we had been invited to start a birth center inside the existing clinic of a general practitioner. At that time, we did not own a vehicle ourselves, so we arranged with the local health center to call for their ambulance if needed.

One night we had a woman with a long, difficult labor and decided we should begin the process of transferring her to the hospital, which was more than three hours away on the other side of the island. We called the number we had been given for ambulance transport, only to be told that the vehicle could not come because it was after midnight. Surprised, I asked what difference the time made, and the reply came that the only available driver was usually drunk after midnight.

We quickly made other arrangements, but it was a hard lesson. Hearing my story, my dad donated money to buy a van that we converted into an ambulance, and from that point forward, we have made it a priority to ensure that every one of our birth centers has its own dedicated ambulance. A good plan anticipates the details you hope you never face, and this is true in all settings.

Birth Preparedness and Complication Readiness (BP/CR) is a framework designed by Jhpiego, a Johns Hopkins University affiliate that is dedicated to improving care for women and families worldwide, to recognize and reduce delays in maternity care. This is a strategy that saves untold lives through simple preparation leading to prevention of delays. The idea is simple but powerful: If families and communities are prepared for birth and also ready for the possibility of complications, they are far more likely to seek skilled care in time. Too often, mothers and babies suffer not because help does not exist, but because it is delayed or thought to be inaccessible. BP/CR addresses the three deadly delays by encouraging proactive planning.

Families are guided to plan where the mother will give birth, who will accompany her, and how to reach skilled care if it becomes necessary. They are instructed on recognizing danger signs during pregnancy. They are encouraged to set aside money for transportation and possible hospital fees, to arrange for a blood donor in case one might be needed, and to identify a decision-maker who can act quickly in an emergency. The BP/CR framework calls for awareness that we all have to work together to improve transportation, communication, and coordination with health facilities so that the pathway to higher-level care is smooth rather than filled with obstacles and delays.

For midwives, this framework provides a way to prepare in advance to manage complications so that if sudden danger arises, it does not catch anyone off guard and woefully unprepared. Birth preparedness directly reduces the first two delays in the three-delays model by helping families recognize warning signs and make sure transport, funds, and decision-making are already in place. Complication readiness helps reduce the third delay by ensuring that health facilities and providers are alert, equipped, and prepared to receive patients in need, any time of the day or night. These frameworks give us a strategic approach: fewer delays, faster response, and better outcomes for mothers and babies.

HIGH-RESOURCE COUNTRY PLAN

A few models that have emerged in recent years in the United States of America resemble this concept. The Home to Hospital Transfer Guidelines, created by the Home Birth Summit, is a wonderful resource hammered out between obstetricians, pediatricians, community midwives, and emergency medical services. Another one is Step Up Together, with their modular drill kits to plan, run, and debrief a drill for a birth emergency that involves a transfer from a community-based setting to a hospital. In Washington state, Smooth Transitions is an initiative aimed at improving communication and enhancing collaboration between community midwives and hospital-based providers. There are other smaller, community-based programs that encourage providers to cooperate rather than work at odds with each other, and I commend anyone doing this hard work proactively.

The goal of being prepared for the worst is to create a framework of collaboration across perceived boundaries, establishing vital links for communication, consultation, and referral among maternity care practitioners in different settings. Babies are born in all kinds of settings: at home, in community birth centers, in small hospitals, and in tertiary-level medical centers and teaching hospitals. A small number of mothers and newborns will require specialist-level care. When we expect the unexpected and plan for possible birth complications and emergencies in advance, it is a smart strategy that is bound to lead to better outcomes, increased satisfaction with care, and decreased practitioner liability.

SAFE MOTHERHOOD INITIATIVE FRAMEWORK

The final framework I will mention is one dear to my heart, one we have used from the beginning of Mercy In Action's global work. It is the World Health Organization's Safe Motherhood Initiative, launched in 1987. This initiative was one of the first global frameworks to call attention to maternal mortality as a public health crisis and to outline strategies for reducing preventable deaths. I cannot emphasize enough what this meant to all of us doing this work in the 1980s when it came out. Finally, maternal death was named as a preventable injustice instead of an inevitable result of poverty, and a strategy was presented. Since Mercy In Action's beginnings as a nonprofit were in that same decade, we aligned our work from the start with the vision of the Safe Motherhood Initiative.

The Safe Motherhood Initiative emphasized improving access to skilled midwifery care, ensuring emergency obstetric services, and addressing the social determinants of health that put women at risk of dying during pregnancy, childbirth, and postpartum. Until I read it for the first time, I honestly did not know that midwives were so badly needed everywhere in the world.

Safe motherhood, along with newborn survival, has been a guiding framework for how we have trained midwives, designed programs, and delivered care in low-resource settings for decades. By combining the focus on survival with our belief that the mother and baby can thrive through an empowering birth experience, our vision and strategy were clarified early on: to protect natural birth while preventing complications and responding quickly when emergencies arise. Our provision of maternity care, delivered with kindness, compassion, and respect, with an emphasis on underserved populations, has achieved excellent outcomes and demonstrated that frameworks are vital to achieving our goals of safe motherhood and child survival.

MIDWIVES ARE NOT ALONE

Recently, the World Health Organization launched a new resource for maternity care providers. As I was putting the finishing touches on this chapter, I was honored to be asked to share our Mercy In Action model alongside dedicated researchers from Geneva as they rolled out the *Compendium on Respectful Maternal and Newborn Care.*

Sharing a webinar stage with women from WHO and ICI, who have devoted their careers to making birth safer and more respectful in countries around the world, reminded me again that midwives do not carry this work alone. I am fortunate to belong to a whole community of public health experts and maternal and newborn health scientists who support our work. These non-midwives are vital contributors to the work midwives do.

I am so thankful for Michelle Skaer Therrien, Executive Director of the International Childbirth Initiative, who is deeply passionate about supporting birth facilities that offer the 12 Steps. I am privileged to know and work beside doctors like André LaLonde from Canada and Carlos Fuchtner from Bolivia, who work tirelessly to promote ICI among their obstetrician peers around the world. Eugene Declercq, professor at Boston University School of Public Health and creator of Birth by the Numbers, has provided invaluable research on maternity outcomes that informs our work.

A whole network of doulas, childbirth educators, and lactation consultants framed the first drafts of mother-friendly documents dating back to the Coalition for Improving Maternity Services in the 1990s, friends like Rae Davies and Debra Pascali-Bonaro who continue to push for better birth to this day. Educators like Rebecca Dekker from the USA, a nurse who founded Evidence Based Birth, and Toni Harman from the UK, filmmaker and founder of the Microbirth initiative, also play a key role in helping birth providers translate evidence into practice. Dynamic advocates such as Christy Turlington Burns of Every Mother Counts have brought visibility, funding, and legitimacy to maternal health and midwifery care on a global scale. Midwives are not alone in this fight, and we never were.

FRAMEWORKS AND STRATEGY

Each of the frameworks we have discussed aligns with my vision of strategic midwifery rooted in our core purpose of improving health and healthcare for vulnerable mothers and newborns everywhere. Each provides a lens through which we can evaluate and strengthen the care we offer. All have provided us with valuable insights, from which my team and the people we serve have greatly benefited.

As they are both visionary and practical, models and frameworks hold us accountable to the highest standards of care for mothers, babies, and families. They call us to act as our best selves as birth providers. Strategic midwifery is not only about skill in the moment, but about choosing to see the bigger picture and to work within systems that guide us toward safety, respect, and justice at all times. Taken together, the frameworks and models described in this chapter have created a firm foundation on which Mercy In Action continues to build our excellent outcomes.

In the next two chapters, I will describe some of the creative innovations my team and I have imagined, developed, and implemented to further strengthen our strategic midwifery work.

PAUSE FOR REFLECTION

Are you using any identifiable frameworks currently in your birth setting, and how do you communicate those to your clients or patients? What is your plan to help everyone in your care receive just-right maternity care that avoids too much too soon and too little too late? In what ways can you see it benefiting your practice to implement the 12 Steps to Safe and Respectful MotherBaby-Family Maternity Care of the International Childbirth Initiative?

6

CREATIVE INNOVATIONS

Creativity is thinking up new things. Innovation is doing new things.

— THEODORE LEVITT

THE VISION FOR SOME OF OUR MOST SIGNIFICANT BIRTH INNOVATIONS came to me in the most ordinary of settings. In this chapter, we will explore several innovations that we have envisioned and implemented within Mercy In Action, examining the role that creativity plays in shaping a birth culture that is relevant and responsive to the needs of childbearing families and healthcare teams alike.

ORDINARY MOMENTS, EXTRAORDINARY IDEAS

A spark of an idea came to me once while I sat on the edge of a fountain with my son Zak, not long after he returned from deployment with the US Air Force. We were discussing capacity building in our Philippine setting when he casually mentioned something the military uses called an After Action Review. I stopped him mid-story.

"Wait," I said, "tell me that again." As he spoke, I felt a light switch flip on in my mind. I could see clearly how this simple yet structured debrief he was describing could be woven into midwifery, providing a concrete way to pause and reflect after each birth, thereby becoming better at our similarly high-stakes job.

One idea that positively shifted our culture of postpartum care came while my husband Scott and I were on a long road trip across the United States, driving from California on the West Coast to Connecticut in the East. I was in the passenger seat with miles of open road stretched out before us, the hum of the tires creating space for my thoughts to wander. Somewhere along that journey, an idea began to take shape: a post-birth scoring chart that could help midwives individualize follow up care for mothers after delivery in a more targeted way.

Another time, weary after a string of long labors, our midwives were discussing the danger of fatigue. We all knew how exhaustion can cloud judgment until it feels like thinking through fog. I was recalling a practice I had seen while attending a home birth in the Netherlands years before. Out of those conversations, my son Ian sketched a simple workflow diagram to help keep every midwife alert and vigilant, even when the hours on duty stretched long. That sketch became a method for defining roles during labor and delivery to safeguard the well-being of the healthcare team as well as the mother and baby.

Shortly after, while I was on a tour of a ship in Subic Bay, the captain mentioned the danger of everyone rushing to one side of the boat if something caught their attention, as it would cause the whole vessel to tilt precariously. The insight I gained on that ship's bridge ultimately provided us with a new way to teach balance, teamwork, and clarity under pressure, and tied perfectly into the flowchart we were creating at the time. Two problems got rolled into one solution that we have used ever since.

These moments of inspiration remind me that innovation is not what we often think it is. It is rarely the work of a lone genius sitting in an office. More often, it comes as a flash of insight arising from ordinary situations we encounter in life. Innovation takes root when imagination meets a genuine need, and when an idea becomes compelling enough to move us toward action. The hard work of turning ideas and insights into something usable is the very essence of visionary and strategic midwifery, rooted in purpose and mission. It is not leaving outcomes to chance but shaping them through foresight and creativity.

CREATIVITY AT WORK

Over the years, I have watched ideas born within Mercy In Action grow from a seed of inspiration into innovations that reshape the way we serve. Each innovation has been driven by a simple desire to care for people more faithfully and more effectively. While many of these ideas originated with me, they only became a reality through collaboration within our team, and our joint willingness to learn together through trial and error.

Before an idea becomes part of our standard practice, it is tested and refined, training materials are developed, and our entire team is brought on board. Only then is a new idea launched in our birth centers. If it succeeds and leads to improved outcomes, it may be incorporated into our midwifery college curriculum and presented in seminars worldwide as well. The innovations that proved strong over the past half century now form part of the fabric of every birth center we support and every midwifery program we teach. Most of our innovations are designed to be adaptable in any setting, whether high- or low-resource, and have become a key to our success in improving outcomes for mothers and babies.

Of course, nothing we have come up with is truly original. As King Solomon wisely observed, there is nothing new under the sun. What we call innovation is often less about something entirely new and more about interdisciplinary insight, a shift in how we see or explain what has always been there. Much of what we offer is the result of cross-pollination, where ideas long present in other fields are brought into new contexts. We are aware that others have voiced similar truths before us, and no one idea we use is earthshaking on its own. Still and yet, put together, the adaptations and innovations Mercy In Action has created over time make our birth spaces safer, smarter, and more responsive to the needs of mothers, babies, and families. And they have the added benefit of improving working conditions and occupational satisfaction for our midwives.

WHAT IS CREATIVITY?

Before I share the details concerning some of Mercy In Action's more unique innovations for the birth world, let us pause to explore the roots of creativity, because it is there that so many lasting solutions are born. Creativity comes in many forms. While most people associate creativity with the arts, creative ideas are more often realized in everyday work and find expression in innovations that allow us to do something better.

For a midwife attending home births, a touch of creativity is essential. This is what allows us to adapt quickly in each unique home setting. Unlike a birth center or hospital, we do not have the luxury of familiarity with the placement of furniture, supplies, and equipment. Instead, the home birth midwife must improvise at every single labor, organizing supplies from the birth bags we carry in and arranging them in a way that fits the space. At the same time, we must always plan for the unexpected, including how to make a swift egress in case of emergencies, regardless of the type of bedroom, hallway, or doorway we find ourselves in.

Much has been studied and written about the roots of creativity, who possesses it, and how it can be nurtured. One of the latest areas of research on the subject is the study of why most people with ideas don't ever do anything about them. It seems that it takes unusual courage and a high tolerance for risk to act on creative ideas. Acting upon creative urges requires perseverance, resilience, humility, and cooperation with others. These are some of the character traits we can work to develop in our lives that will serve our purpose and lead to better birth outcomes.

Creativity requires another character trait as well, and that is curiosity. Einstein once said, "I have no special talent. I am only passionately curious." Midwives who desire to nurture creative confidence will want to commit to staying curious. Curiosity enhances creative thinking, which in turn complements critical thinking to facilitate more effective problem-solving. Curiosity keeps the mind active, nimble, and able to notice things other people might walk right past.

Creativity is not reserved for a select few; it can be embraced by anyone. Each of us has the ability to ask fresh questions and imagine new solutions. Every child starts out instinctively believing they are creative. As adults, we often seem to lose that confidence along the way. What I know is that creativity in my life is equally a gift and a discipline. It is exciting to tap into my creativity, but doing so often leads to a lot of extra work and a certain amount of stress. I love the process of developing ideas, testing them, and putting them out into the world, yet every time I speak publicly to present new concepts, I need to push past my feelings of vulnerability in doing so. I suppose I am like most people in this; the end result has to feel worth the risk.

How we think affects what we do with our ideas. Stanford professor and psychologist Albert Bandura demonstrated that our belief systems profoundly shape our actions, goals, and perceptions. When people believe they can effect change, they are far more likely to do so. And when they feel their contribution truly matters, they experience greater joy and satisfaction in their work, even when they do get criticized.

For midwives, valuing and nurturing our own creativity may be one of the keys to preventing the burnout that plagues so many in our profession. Dreaming up new solutions to old problems in practical ways is not only appreciated by our clients and patients; it is also life-giving to us. The deep personal satisfaction that comes from bringing creativity into every part of our job may be a factor in our ability to sustain joy in our midwifery work throughout our life course. The opposite is also true. Continuing to complain about the things we could be working on to change will drain our energy.

PURSUING CREATIVITY

Pursuing creativity is not so much a destination as a deliberate journey. Being creative requires more than natural talent, as it also calls upon humility and courage and a number of other character traits. Creativity manifests in both big and small ways, and in unexpected places. We need only to have eyes to see. Matt once told me, "I don't really think of myself as creative," yet when he said that I immediately remembered a moment twenty-plus years ago when we were running Mercy In Action on a tight budget, and he figured out a way to wire a common light switch into our van. That simple fix cost under two dollars and saved us from buying a seventy-five-dollar replacement part at the auto supply store, and it's stuck with me ever since. Sometimes the most creative acts are humble, practical solutions. We don't want to overlook or underestimate those everyday moments of ingenuity that help us do our mission better while spending less money!

UNIQUE BIRTH INNOVATIONS

As we explore some of the Mercy In Action innovations that have become integral to our practice of strategic midwifery, let yourself imagine how you could use them. These ideas, which grew out of real needs in real birth settings, worked so well for us that they became part of the rhythm of every birth center we run. Over the years, we've shared our ideas on how to improve birth outcomes far and wide in articles and seminars, and midwives around the world have reported back to us that they find them useful. As you read, you may find yourself thinking that you too could adapt some of these innovations to your setting.

MERCY IN ACTION'S POST-BIRTH SCORING CHART

Going back to that long cross-country trip I told you about—Scott and I had days on the open road to think and dream as we drove through mountain passes, forests, and wide stretches of plains. One day as we were listening to an audiobook Scott had chosen, my thoughts kept drifting back to the mothers in our care in the Philippines. I was especially preoccupied with the question of providing good postpartum care in a cultural setting where its importance was not yet recognized and where home visits after birth were not common among the midwives.

Postpartum is a sweet and tender time, but also a time of potential danger. It is a season when mothers need special monitoring and nurturing. The immediate days after birth could feel uncertain and unpredictable to anyone, but many of the mothers in our care in the Philippines return home after birth to small shacks without adequate food or sanitation. Knowing that most maternal deaths happen not during pregnancy or labor but in the postpartum period, I kept asking myself, Who might be slipping through the cracks? Who needs more attention than we are giving? How can we continue to care for them after they leave the safe walls of the birth center?

Then something that was said brought my focus back to the audiobook playing through the truck's speakers. The author was Atul Gawande, a renowned medical doctor who thinks beyond conventional boundaries. As Gawande described a surgical scoring system he had developed, he explained how this safety net allowed postoperative care to be personally tailored to each patient recovering from surgery.

Instantly, my mind went to Dr. Virginia Apgar. In 1952, this pioneering anesthesiologist developed a similar scoring system to triage newborn care in the very first moments of life after birth using five key criteria. Before her creation of the now-famous Apgar score, all newborns were treated the same. Her simple scoring system taught birth attendants everywhere to see babies differently and respond to each infant's unique needs at birth. I discovered that Gawande had indeed riffed off Virginia Apgar's idea to create his post-surgical scoring chart. Now I was going to borrow the concept from both of them.

An Assessment Tool Is Born

I wondered what would happen if I created something like the Apgar score for triaging postpartum mothers. A way to quickly assess, personalize, and respond to those individuals who may be at higher risk after birth. A tool that would help us decide who needed extra home visits, who might need to stay a little longer at the birth center, and who was at risk if we departed from their home birth too soon after birth. This score would not be based solely on any one symptom but on a more comprehensive picture.

Getting excited, I grabbed something to write with and started drawing it out. By the time the next truck stop came into view and we pulled over for gas, I had the beginnings of a postpartum scoring chart scribbled in the margins of an old travel brochure. It was a start.

I used five prompts, so each thing could be scored from 0 to 2 and would add up to a perfect score of 10. A score of 10 would indicate that no problems were expected postpartum. I decided to make it a mnemonic around the word *BIRTH*. The letters seemed a good fit to key words from the major causes of maternal mortality and morbidity after birth in our low-resource setting—hemorrhage, infection, obstructed labor, and preeclampsia/eclampsia.

I fiddled with the mnemonic for weeks while we were traveling, and upon my return to the Philippines, I worked with our team to refine the chart. Because everyone trained in maternity care is familiar with the Apgar score, it was easy to explain, and before long, it became a part of how we provided care. I was thrilled to realize how easy it was to deliver more personalized, more responsive, and protective care to mothers in that delicate time after birth.

That's the thing about innovation. Sometimes it's just paying attention to what's been done before and could be revised, or what works in another field and could be repurposed. It's making space for ideas to meet the needs before us.

POST-BIRTH SCORING CHART

FOR POSTPARTUM RISK

Created by Vicki Penwell for Mercy In Action

	Birth Factors	0	1	2	Score
B	Blood pressure at any time in labor or immediate postpartum	< 90/50 or > 140/90	Borderline hypo- or hyper- tension	Within normal range	
I	Infection risk: fever* or frequent internal exams during labor	Fever* or > 7 internal exams	Fever* or 3–7 internal exams	No fever and < 3 internal exams	
R	Repair required for birth canal lacerations	3rd or 4th degree laceration	1st or 2nd degree laceration or episiotomy	No sutures required no lacerations	
T	Time of active labor after 6 cm dilation	> 24 hours	12–24 hours	< 12 hours	
H	Hemorrhage - total blood loss (EBL) at birth & immediate postpartum	> 1,000 cc	500–1,000 cc	< 500 cc	
				Total Score →	

* fever defined as temperature > 100.4° F or 38° C

ANY SCORE OF 0 ON A SINGLE FACTOR, OR A TOTAL SCORE OF ≤ 7, INDICATES NEED FOR SPECIAL POSTPARTUM FOLLOW-UP

Recognition of the Need

The Post-Birth Scoring Chart was developed years before in response to our observations that midwives in the Southeast Asian countries we lived in and visited conduct very few postpartum visits. Some midwives told us they do not do home visits at all, while others expect the woman to come back to their clinic, which often did not happen. Others told us they make home visits in the days after birth sporadically, and when I asked them what might prevent them from doing so, they listed several reasons why they might miss a postpartum home visit. This list included if it was raining, if the patient lived too far away, or if it was a holiday. This was what first alerted us to the realization that postpartum home visits were rarely based on medical need, but rather on convenience and the weather. Granted, weather can be extreme and dangerous in certain parts of the world, but the data suggested a larger issue: failing to account for any extenuating factors that might have occurred at the birth to make the mother more high-risk postpartum.

Even in America, where postpartum care is generally considered to be highly valued by midwives, I conducted an informal study at a few midwife gatherings and found, based on a survey, that most midwives used the same schedule of visits for every postpartum mother, regardless of the circumstances surrounding the birth. Like their Asian counterparts, they also admitted to occasionally skipping a postpartum visit for the same reasons. These factors were random and again not tied to any principles of medical triage.

Criteria

In thinking through what I had discovered about postpartum care being routine at best and often altogether absent, I was struck again by the brilliance of Virginia Apgar's invention. With five simple criteria, she provided the doctors, nurses, and midwives with a way to view each baby as an individual and respond accordingly. Dr. Gawande, looking through the eyes of a surgeon, recognized a similar need to individualize postoperative care, and designed the Surgical Apgar Score.

Drawing from these insights, I began to imagine what a comparable tool might mean for mothers after birth. In developing our Post-Birth Scoring Chart, we wanted to take into account what actually happened during the birth in order to anticipate possible postpartum problems before they occurred.

How It Works

Based on the score obtained before discharge after the birth, we may decide to keep a mother in the birth center a little longer for closer monitoring, or we may increase the frequency of follow-up home visits in the days to come. The chart allows us to personalize the postpartum period and helps us identify who needs extra vigilance. When a low score alerts us to risk, we make it a priority to monitor more often, whether that means staying longer after birth, going out in a storm, rearranging our schedule, or asking a fellow midwife to cover if we are attending another birth and unable to keep a postpartum appointment.

Postpartum Risk Factors

The Post-Birth Scoring Chart is primarily looking for risk factors that could potentially lead to the four most common global causes of maternal mortality and morbidity. During the refinement of our chart, we found data suggesting that these warning signs, observed during labor, delivery, and the immediate postpartum period, were linked to a higher risk of complications and emergencies in the postpartum period, as follows.

B = Blood Pressure

Increased blood pressure is a risk factor for a number of different problems postpartum, with a particularly dangerous complication being the development of preeclampsia and eclampsia. If a woman's blood pressure has gone above 140/90 in labor, she is at risk for a postpartum episode of hypertension, which could be an early warning sign of postpartum preeclampsia or eclampsia. In addition, high blood pressure alone is also a risk for disrupting the placental site clot, leading to secondary (late) postpartum hemorrhage.

Decreased blood pressure could be a sign of shock from blood loss. Anytime the blood pressure in the intrapartum or immediate postpartum period goes below 90/50, the mother is at risk and should be monitored carefully. She is also at risk of fainting if blood pressure is running unnaturally low after birth.

I = Infection

Fever is a universal sign of possible infection. An excess of vaginal exams during labor is a risk factor for infection, with or without ruptured membranes. Every vaginal exam increases the risk of infection, even when done with sterile technique, as the gloved fingers can move bacteria from the lower vaginal vault higher up where it can get a foothold in the reproductive organs.

One difficulty we have encountered in reporting is that many midwives only chart vaginal exams conducted in the first stage of labor, but in the second stage, they may put their gloved fingers in multiple times to check how far down the baby is descending, or they may push on the pelvic floor as the presenting part descends. Those are all considered vaginal exams in labor and should be added up for the post-birth risk scoring.

R = Repairs

Lacerations or tears of the birth canal, including episiotomy, increase the risk of infection. Also, while lacerations are a known risk for infection, they could also be a risk for hemorrhage if they bleed excessively before being sutured. The best healing after birth occurs with minimal or no tearing of the reproductive tract.

T = Time

Length of labor is something else we measure. A longer labor is not in itself a risk factor in most cases, but we are watching for signs of obstructed labor. Even if it eventually resolves, it may have exhausted the mother to the point of her being at higher risk of hemorrhage or infection. Although it is rare these days for anyone to die of obstructed labor in rich countries, it is still a common occurrence in low-resource nations. There are other problems brought on by excessively long labor, for example, experiencing unrelenting pain for hours on end can temporarily weaken the immune system, leaving a postpartum mother more vulnerable to infection. A difficult labor that is finally resolved is associated with maternal exhaustion that can lead to uterine atony, the most common cause of postpartum hemorrhage. A long labor is often associated with more total vaginal exams as well. Long labors have a higher likelihood of needing to wrestle out a shoulder dystocia or use manipulation to bring out an after-coming head in a breech presentation. Any manual manipulation of the baby at birth has been shown to result in increased risk of infection and hemorrhage for the mother.

H = Hemorrhage

Losing too much blood at birth is a problem that can carry consequences in the postpartum period. While not everyone experiences the effects of blood loss in the same way, losing too much blood is harmful, whether it occurs immediately after birth or gradually over the hours that follow. If a patient has a low score on this indicator, she is closer to the line where she could go into shock postpartum from more bleeding. We also know that losing a lot of blood at birth can increase the risk for postpartum infection.

Ongoing Feedback

Mercy In Action has used our chart in thousands of births, and it definitely makes our decisions on postpartum care more scientific as we evaluate each individual mother's risk. The idea is that no one gets less than the standard number of visits postpartum, but some mothers get more, which is what individualized maternity care needs to look like to be truly safe. Our Post-Birth Scoring Chart now helps maternity care providers everywhere to consciously consider what constitutes risks in the postpartum period, based on what happened during the birth, and provide extra attention as appropriate. Before someone leaves our immediate care after birth, we first determine what risk factors may complicate the postpartum period.

We have run studies demonstrating that it is an effective tool for identifying postpartum mothers who require closer monitoring. We have also taught this scoring system around the world and always ask midwives who take our training to test it in their own facilities and give us feedback.

Amanda, a former student of Mercy In Action, studied it as her capstone project for a master's degree in maternal-child health systems. She suggested that we might want to consider adding an *S* for support to the end to make it BIRTHS and add the risk factors for the level of existing mental health support, as there is evidence that we can prevent or minimize postpartum depression with better professional and family support after birth. There are also advantages to maintaining our chart in the simple five-item format, which is familiar to everyone who already uses the Apgar scoring tool. The point is that the chart is adaptable.

MERCY IN ACTION'S NEWBORN HAT CLASSIFICATION SYSTEM

Every baby needs three things at birth: warmth, mother's milk, and love. In order to have the best chance to survive and thrive, babies should be skin-to-skin in their mother's arms immediately after birth, held close to the breast where they can start taking in colostrum, the first milk. Ninety-six percent of babies born in our Mercy In Action sponsored birth centers begin breastfeeding within the first hour of life, the time recommended by experts and endorsed by the World Health Organization. Babies born after an unmedicated labor and birth almost always display strong instinctive feeding behaviors and will frequently begin breastfeeding even sooner—many of ours begin within the first fifteen minutes—when mother and baby are kept together in a calm, quiet, undisturbed environment.

In Mercy In Action birth centers, we encourage women to give birth in positions that are safest and most comfortable for both mother and baby. Positions that are upright or side-lying allow the sacrum the flexibility to move freely, creating maximum space in the birth canal for the baby to emerge without distress. After birth, our midwives do not place the baby onto the mother's abdomen; instead, we wait for the mother to reach for her own baby. As she gathers her newborn into her arms, her natural instinct is to bring the baby to her breast.

All vital signs are carefully monitored during the first hour after birth while the baby stays skin to skin in the mother's arms. Respiration, heart rate, and temperature are assessed without disturbing bonding or the baby's first breastfeed. If the room is warm, the baby does not need a hat right away. Many midwives advocate that a baby's head stay uncovered in the first hour after birth (known as the Golden Hour) so that mothers can smell and kiss their baby's head.

A Hat Color Is Chosen

At about one hour after birth, or sooner if the room is not really warm, the baby is given a hat, and the color of that hat corresponds to the baby's clinical classification. This simple visual system helps caregivers quickly recognize whether the baby needs routine monitoring (green), closer observation and more frequent monitoring (yellow), or continuous observation because the baby may require transfer to a higher-level medical facility (red). Babies in the red hat category are monitored continuously until their condition stabilizes or they are safely transferred to advanced care.

Newborn Hat Classification

GREEN	YELLOW	RED
• Normal vitals • Normal weight • Normal delivery • Clear amniotic fluid • Cried at birth • APGAR score 8 or above • Latched and nursed in first hour	• Meconium staining or premature rupture of membranes in labor • Needed help to start breathing at birth • Premature or postmature • APGAR score 7 or below • Abnormal respiratory patterns • Any abnormal vital sign • Minor birth defect noted • Mother tested positive for GBS or had signs of GBS infection in labor • Mother tested positive for hep B or HIV • Mother tested positive for any sexual transmitted disease • Not latched yet at one hour old • Low birth weight (less than 2500 grams) • Birth injury • Cardiac irregularities • Pale, cyanotic, or gray color • Abnormal cry • Lethargy and low muscle tone	• Major birth defect noted • Respiratory distress • Seizures • Jaundice at birth • Any neonatal distress not responsive to interventions

This color-coded system provides an immediate visual assessment during the first hours after birth, whether the baby is being monitored in a birth facility or after a home delivery. The baby's color designation is also recorded in the chart and helps guide care during the days and weeks following birth.

We have found this system to be very effective for training midwives, nurses, and aides because it provides staff with an immediate visual reminder of each baby's risk level during the newborn transition period. If special hats are not available, the same color-coding system can be used with stickers on the birth room door or by marking the chart with the appropriate color. However, the hats make it especially easy to recognize at a glance when a baby requires closer attention based on risk factors at birth.

Colored hats help everyone remember not to treat all newborns alike in the hours after birth. This color-coded hat system, like the post-birth scoring chart for mothers, helps us remember to monitor vital signs more often if there were risk factors at birth. It helps us live out our value of giving individualized, personalized care to each unique mother and baby in our care after birth, in order to help them achieve the best outcome possible.

MERCY IN ACTION'S MOTHER-MIDWIFE / BABY-MIDWIFE WORKFLOW

Fatigue from long stretches on the job is one of the greatest challenges midwives face, and it significantly increases the risk of mistakes. Research shows that 17–19 hours without sleep impairs judgment as much as a blood alcohol level of 0.05%, and 20–24 hours without sleep is equivalent to 0.10%, well over the legal driving limit. Just as exhaustion makes drivers slow to notice and react to roadway hazards, it can also dull a midwife's ability to think clearly when assessing risks and responding to birth emergencies. In birth work, where quick decisions can mean life or death, fatigue is not a badge of honor, it is a liability.

Caring well for mothers and babies requires systems that can help prevent such extreme exhaustion, in much the same way that the aviation system keeps pilots from flying when tired. The Three Delays framework I described in the previous chapter reminds us that we must stay sharp in order to recognize potential problems early, as it is known that fatigue can cause poor judgment that leads to delays.

Another danger we face was highlighted to me during that tour I mentioned of a ship in our local harbor. It is obvious yet vital to remind midwives that there are always a minimum of two people at each birth who may both require skilled emergency assistance simultaneously. A delayed reaction can occur when all attention is focused on one patient, much like passengers rushing to one side of a boat, causing it to capsize and endanger everyone. Both mother and baby deserve vigilant care simultaneously; we need to be careful to avoid capsizing their boat, metaphorically speaking. The following story I heard from a midwife friend illustrates this point.

Caught on Video

As a child, Rachel Mast remembers watching the video recording of her own birth. After entering the midwifery profession, Rachel asked her mother if she could watch it again, but this time she saw something she had never noticed. In the video, she realized her mother had begun to hemorrhage after her birth, and the midwives present rushed to care for her. But as Rachel looked closer, she realized something chilling. The baby in the video—Rachel herself—had stopped breathing while pressed against her mother's chest. She saw her body turning blue. This went unnoticed, as all attention was on her bleeding mother. She told me she watched, horrified, wanting to yell through the screen, "Check the baby!" Eventually someone noticed the baby, asked, "Is she breathing?" and quickly snatched her up and began clearing her airway, and Rachel heard her newborn self give a gasp and then a cry.

Obviously, Rachel lived to tell this story, but it illustrates the point of what can happen unintentionally when everyone is rushing to care for one patient in need. I have also witnessed the reverse situation: Silent postpartum bleeding is pooling onto the sheets, overlooked while everyone in the room focused on reviving a newborn, counting off the rhythm of resuscitation while oblivious to a crisis unfolding for the other patient in the room. Because postpartum hemorrhage is silent and painless, even the mother may not realize what is happening, distracted as she is by concern for her newborn. The vigilance must extend to both mother and baby at once. Both deserve equally attentive care in those vulnerable moments after birth.

Two Roles

To address these dangers, my son Ian created what we call our Mother-Midwife / Baby-Midwife Workflow, to be used by two or more midwives at a birth. This recognizes that every birth involves two patients, the mother and the newborn, so there should always be at least two trained birth attendants present. Sometimes both the mother and baby need help at the same time. This scenario is more common than one might think, because situations that can cause a baby to need resuscitation at birth (for instance, shoulder dystocia, breech, long labor, or precipitous labor) are also risk factors for hemorrhaging in the mother.

How It Works

With this system the two midwives decide in advance which of them will serve primarily as the mother-midwife and which will serve primarily as the baby-midwife. Of course, they are not locked into these roles; they are at the same bedside, after all, and can be fluid to respond as needed. The important thing is that in the event of a complication or an emergency, this designation in advance prevents delays or duplication of effort as each midwife remains focused on her own patient, while also being free to lend a hand to the other midwife as needed.

Besides preventing confusion, this model significantly addresses the common problem of all the attendants at a birth being tired at the same time. The mother-midwife is the first to arrive on the scene when a labor call comes in and monitors maternal well-being throughout the first stage of labor. The early stage of labor can take hours and is often in the middle of the night, but the exhausted midwife knows help is on the way around the time second-stage labor is approaching. This help arrives in the form of the baby-midwife, who is rested and ready to put fresh eyes on the situation. She reviews the chart and helps get everything set up for the birth.

With two fully trained midwives now in the room as the baby emerges, the mother-midwife manages the delivery of the baby and placenta and keeps a close eye on maternal vital signs in the time immediately after birth to quickly identify potential complications. The baby-midwife assumes responsibility for the newborn's transition, assisting with the first breaths if needed, supporting the start of breastfeeding, and monitoring the vital signs of the baby in the first crucial moments after birth. If both mother and baby experience a complication at the same time, both patients receive immediate, skilled attention from their designated midwife without time wasted by confusion over roles.

Changing of the Guard

Once the birth is complete and the MotherBaby dyad is safely tucked in and bonding, the baby-midwife assumes responsibility for the postpartum watch while the mother-midwife can step away and either go home or go to lie down and rest. This feature of the model is vital because without it both midwives might reach the moment of birth already exhausted and risk lowering their guard afterward in the immediate postpartum period. Yet in those first few hours after birth, mothers need support with establishing breastfeeding, getting up to urinate, and later, eating and showering, and babies require vigilant observation as they make the delicate transition from fetal to postnatal circulation and adjust to life outside the womb. With this model, the hours immediately following birth are now covered by a wide-awake midwife who was not up all night.

This concept of sharing responsibility does not rely on a system of hierarchy. As long as both midwives are equally trained to perform either role, they simply decide in advance who does what and trade off at the next labor. In our birth centers, we have a magnet board where we can see at a glance the names of the two midwives on call and which role they will assume when the next labor arrives.

We are sometimes asked how this could work for an independent home birth midwife who only brings a student apprentice or a birth assistant. In that case, the student or assistant would be designated for the baby and should be certified in neonatal resuscitation. And roles will need to be modified to ensure compliance with the professional scope of practice, given that this is intended for use by two fully qualified midwives. Student midwives are never allowed to be on their own without a supervising preceptor in the room.

Decision Tree

If you want to make this concept visual and practical as a checklist of sorts, you can draw the duties side by side as a sequence of events common in a delivery. In that way, it can also serve as a decision tree, showing the flow of duties of the mother-midwife and the baby-midwife. This is the part that can be personalized to your setting so nothing is overlooked in the moment.

This concept is strategic and practical when there are two midwives practicing together. Midwives appreciate that this system takes into consideration the needs of the birth attendants, as concern for respecting and caring for the providers is one of the steps outlined in the ICI. This model minimizes fatigue and helps mitigate burnout in the midwifery workforce. It avoids the "all eyes on one patient" trap and ensures that both mother and baby receive the full measure of care they deserve. It removes hierarchy and can act as a simple checklist for who does what. This model adapts easily to home births, birth centers, and hospital birth teams. It also works well in training environments where apprentice midwives are assigned to roles under supervision, and they focus on learning their duties in just one role at a time. We even use this model during simulation drills.

Now let us turn our attention to one of the most significant habits we have built within our Mercy In Action culture to improve outcomes as well as strengthen morale and a sense of control among our midwives. It's called After Action Review.

MERCY IN ACTION'S AFTER ACTION REVIEW

Humility is admitting we have more to learn. The seed of an idea to run with this concept took root in me one day while talking to my eldest son about his experiences serving in Afghanistan and Iraq during the years of conflict. Zak mentioned how his military team would gather to debrief, and my curiosity was piqued. I asked for details. He explained how soldiers and those who supported them would sit down together after every mission to go over what went well, what went wrong, and what they could do better next time. They use a very structured format known as an After Action Review.

I couldn't stop thinking about how this structured approach could be adapted for midwifery. It struck me that the intensity, urgency, and danger involved in a delivery complication share some similarities with those found in combat situations. Lives are at stake. Communication is critical. Things are happening fast. Equipment must function, and every team member has to be alert, prepared, and working together. I decided it would be beneficial if midwives could set aside a few moments after a birth to ask what went well, what went wrong, and what could be improved. It made perfect sense to bring this kind of intentional reflective debrief into the world of birth.

A Formal Review

I went to bed that night with my head full of ideas and began working out a midwifery adaptation. This would be something that could take us beyond the random chat or occasional debrief that midwives may do after an interesting or harrowing birth. It would be more immediate than a peer review, and much more personal. Most importantly, if done correctly, it would lead to actionable points and improvements that we could implement immediately. I hoped it would also help build self-awareness and improve our team dynamics.

It wasn't long until I had adapted the concept and written up what it would look like for our birth teams to begin adopting. After working out the kinks with our leaders, I began sharing the concept in our birth centers. I knew that to be effective it had to be consistent, and it would take a concerted effort to get everyone into this new habit. At the time we launched, I was overseeing a birth center in Manila that averaged one hundred births per month. We had four birth teams that each had a caseload of approximately twenty-five births each month, or almost one per day. To ask them to add one more thing to a schedule like that was a big ask, so I had to convince them it was going to be a positive change.

We held an all-team meeting to institute the After Action Review into our practice, and I acknowledged how hard it would be to build new habits when everyone was already working so hard. I asked each birth team to commit to thirty days straight of never missing holding an After Action Review after a birth. We would determine after this trial period if we would continue or reevaluate.

One of our young midwives spoke up during the meeting and asked with a grin, "What will you do to us if we forget?" I laughed and said, "You can think up your own punishment." That lightened the mood in the room, and soon everyone was laughing as each team began inventing their own consequence for forgetting, most of them far tougher than anything I would have suggested. From that day forward, no one missed an After Action Review for the next one hundred births, and a new habit was born. It did not take long for all our midwives to embrace the practice as something constructive, and once it was a habit, it was easy to do. Now we cannot imagine working without it, in any setting.

The After Action Review is not about any one individual but is always about the bigger picture, encompassing all birth team members, their equipment, and the physical space in which they are working. It includes the primary attendants present (midwives, doctors, or nurses), their assistants and support team, the birth supplies and equipment they used, and interactions with the environment, such as the birth room or facility in general. It also could include vehicles if a transport became necessary.

How It Works

The simple review centers on three foundational questions:

1. What did we do right, or what went well and why?
2. What did we do poorly, or what went wrong and why?
3. What can be improved, or what can we do better next time?

These questions help us notice the strengths we want to sustain while also identifying the areas that need improvement. These prompts promote professional growth for the entire birth team in a safe and supportive manner.

Ideally, the After Action Review takes place shortly after the birth, once the mother and baby are stable, while the entire birth team is still gathered and the details are fresh in everyone's minds. The setting should allow for privacy, away from the family but close enough to be convenient and allow for intermittent monitoring of the MotherBaby. Most After Action Reviews can be completed in ten or fifteen minutes, though they may need to be longer after a difficult or traumatic event. The important thing is to make space for everyone to participate honestly, with equal respect for each voice. This means allowing time for everyone to share insights without regard to hierarchy. With an After Action Review, every birth becomes a chance to learn, to strengthen our team, and to serve the next family even better.

The review itself should always begin with the good points, what went well and why, so that best practices are recognized and are more likely to be repeated. This step is crucial because I have found that, over time, midwives can start forgetting to do the right things if these practices are not reinforced.

Next comes the harder but necessary question of what went wrong and why. This is the part that takes courage and honesty. No one likes to discover after a birth that something preventable went wrong, even if it is a minor issue, but this is how we improve and avoid making the same mistakes again in future births.

Finally, the group identifies what could be improved and how. Asking "why" and "how" often reveals the root cause of a problem, but the facilitator must guide the discussion away from blame and toward growth by asking questions like "What will we do differently next time?" An After Action Review should always end with concrete action points and a plan to quickly act on them. These may be recommendations for repairing or replacing broken equipment, arranging an in-service training to strengthen a weak skill, or reinforcing strategies that worked especially well.

When this process becomes part of the culture, the whole birth team benefits. Midwives, students, and staff gain confidence and skills, and mothers and babies receive safer, more thoughtful care. Everybody wins.

Living the After Action Review Results

The greatest benefit of incorporating After Action Reviews into your midwifery practice comes from applying the lessons learned to future births, transports, or other events in which the midwives and team are involved together. By allowing the After Action Review to guide your future decisions on policies to create, in-service training to schedule, readings to assign, or plans to allow your student to go to the next level of responsibility, you are practicing a form of evidence-based preparation and are building a strong foundation for future excellence.

The Role of Humility

Here we return to my premise that inner character work impacts our outer results. There is no way you can do an After Action Review well without humility. Humility allows us to learn, because we can let go of the illusion that we know it all, even when we are the leader or have been doing this birth work a long time. Humility helps us ask for help when we need it and listen to others around us with open hearts.

Bringing the spirit of After Action Review into your culture is about paying attention to detail, admitting when we're wrong, and being open to change so we can achieve better outcomes. Humility toward our peers and students fosters a culture where learning is safe and failure is not the end of the story.

A few years ago, a young midwife new to our team made a mistake during a birth. In the intensity of the moment, something important slipped past her. When it came to light during our After Action Review, she became defensive and agitated. At first, she deflected blame and tried to minimize the oversight by pointing out that no harm had come of the mistake. She justified her error by stating that she was distracted by the laboring woman's intense expressions of pain during the transition phase. But as the other midwives in the room gently pressed without shaming, her demeanor began to shift. With tears in her eyes, she admitted that she had been caught in the trap of time distortion that can happen in the intensity of labor, as well as being caught in the trap of pride that can lead to denial. She began to willingly participate in the After Action Review process, realizing it was not a judgment on her as a person but a means to enable her to improve at what she was passionate about—helping mothers give birth safely. She later told us that the incident had been transformational in her growth as a midwife.

A Tool for Processing

By turning our experiences into opportunities for growth, After Action Review shifts the focus from shame to learning and from blame to accountability. It gives us a way to remember the good and improve the not-so-good. This tool not only sharpens skills, it also shapes character, ensuring that all of us become ever more capable, compassionate, and resilient in the work we do. It is a gift to be able to learn from our mistakes and make fewer mistakes going forward, but it is a difficult gift to accept. We need After Action Review because we have lives in our hands and the stakes are high.

Because of the support structure involved, if done right, the After Action Review could even be an important factor in helping birth attendants to process trauma and see the big picture. Newer research in healthcare settings indicates that greater job control among midwives, which involves the ability to analyze and influence how work is done, is closely linked to higher job satisfaction even under heavy workloads and mental stress.

Disaster Response

After adapting the After Action Review for midwifery, I discovered that many non-military groups have also adapted it for their own unique purposes. When we faced a steep learning curve in disaster response after Typhoon Haiyan/Yolanda struck the Philippines in 2013, I found out that After Action Reviews are also common after major disasters. In fact, After Action Reviews following Hurricane Katrina in America and the 2010 earthquake in Haiti led to new international protocols for emergency communication. One quote from a disaster agency summed it up best: "Without an After Action Review, you keep learning your lessons the hard way."

Achieving a good outcome during a disaster or birth emergency is not just about doing things right; it's also about creating space to do things better next time. When we pause to reflect, to ask what worked, what didn't and why, we make room for creative growth. Learning and improving in this way becomes a key strategy for achieving better results.

Our self-reflective After Action Reviews have become an integral part of our culture, deeply embedded in our midwifery provision of care. Today, After Action Reviews are woven throughout Mercy In Action birth centers and in our college curriculum. We have been sharing the concept in our continuing education seminars, and I have written about it for midwifery journals. During one year's Virtual International Day of the Midwife, I presented on how it can be used for training student midwives in translating theory to practice. I often hear from midwives all over the world who now use it routinely in their practices and love it.

CREATIVE TEAMWORK

No one achieves excellent birth outcomes alone. It is always good to remember how much of our success depends on the close, collaborative work of many. All of the innovations we either created or adapted for our use in Mercy In Action came about because our team identified a need, envisioned a response, and then collaborated to develop a useful tool, model, program, or framework. All these innovations have been tested in our clinical settings for years. At this point in time, the innovations in this chapter have been duplicated and scaled up by other midwives and birth professionals who have adopted our models and are now using them in various birth settings around the world.

I believe that when we act on our creative ideas out of a desire to serve others, it can make a powerful difference. In the next chapter, we will continue our survey of unique Mercy In Action adaptations, innovations, and approaches to the delivery of maternity care and midwifery education by looking at mindsets.

PAUSE FOR REFLECTION

HOW DO YOU CREATE SPACE IN YOUR DAILY PRACTICE FOR IMAGINATION AND PROBLEM-SOLVING? WHAT CHALLENGES IN BIRTH WORK HAVE STIRRED YOU TO THINK DIFFERENTLY OR FIND A NEW APPROACH? HAVE YOU TURNED YOUR IDEAS INTO INNOVATIONS THAT MAKE BIRTH BETTER IN SOME WAY?

7
MINDSET IN MOTION

The place God calls you to is the place where your deep gladness and the world's deep hunger meet.

— FREDERICK BUECHNER

IMAGINE IF MIDWIVES WERE KNOWN NOT ONLY FOR MIDWIFING THE SAFE birth of babies, but also for midwifing better systems of providing maternity care. Just as we tend to mothers and babies with patience and skill, we could also begin to midwife the birth of new ideas, giving them time to grow and guiding them through challenges. We could be delivering fresh approaches and stimulating creativity in each other. In this way, midwifery could become not only the sacred work of assisting in bringing children into the world, but also the calling to birth new and better practices that improve health for mothers, babies, and families everywhere. The mission of the visionary midwife is nothing short of changing birth culture for the better!

Dr. Anshu Banerjee at the World Health Organization wrote, "Expanding and investing in midwifery models of care is one of the most effective strategies to improve maternal and newborn health globally." The WHO has recently called for the expansion of midwifery in every country and released implementation guidance on transitioning hospitals and birthing facilities to the midwifery model of care.

Midwives are central to positive change, yet many carry low self-esteem shaped by a world that has long overlooked and misunderstood their work. I like Misty Copeland's attitude: As the first Black principal ballerina at the American Ballet Theatre, she overcame significant barriers and said that at some point she had to stop listening to the naysayers, because there is more reward in taking a risk than in listening to people who do not understand the mission.

When we set aside self-doubt and choose the courage to create new ways of doing things, innovations find room to grow. I have seen this repeatedly as our team has turned simple ideas into meaningful actions, and our mindsets have transformed our ability to serve well in all maternity care situations, whether low-risk, high-risk, or in-between. That is why this chapter will focus on mindsets and why understanding how the human brain functions is key to our success in achieving good outcomes in birth.

MIDWIFE AS A VERB

Years ago, I began using the word *midwife* in a more creative way, as a verb rather than just a title, hoping it might help people outside the profession understand the heart of what we are all about. For me, it became a way of describing all that we midwives do in a single word that could be conjugated to express action. I began saying things like, "I was out last night midwifing a birth," or "I have midwifed over 3,500 births in my lifetime." It felt right, because being a midwife is not static; it is active, ongoing work that entails both skill and service, and involves much more than our language typically conveys when we describe our work.

Language around the role of a midwife often feels incomplete to me, and is complicated further by general disagreement over terms. To say we "deliver" babies fell out of fashion in the United States decades ago, since technically it is the mother who delivers her own baby, but midwives in many parts of the world still use that phrasing. Other midwives favor the word *catch* to describe their work, as in, "I caught a baby last night," or "I am a baby-catcher." The problem with the word *catch* is that in the empowerment model of birth that we advocate for in Mercy In Action, the midwives are hands-off in a normal delivery. The baby slips onto a clean pad beneath a squatting or kneeling mother, who is upright and in her own power. In this methodology the mother is the one to pick up her own baby and bring it to her breast after birth, with no one actually needing to catch or deliver the baby.

Other phrases such as, "I assist at births," or "I attend births," diminish the true role of midwives, who guide and educate through the pregnancy, carefully monitor through long hours of labor, and occasionally manage birth complications and emergencies in spectacular fashion.

When we use the word *midwife* as a verb, it encompasses the entirety of our work within the midwifery model of care. It spans the spectrum of experiences involved in maternity care and also covers the occasions when we facilitate transfer to higher care, even if that birth ends in a cesarean. This way of speaking also honors the contribution of every midwife in the room, each playing a vital role and carrying part of the responsibility, whether they are the one to "catch" or "deliver" the baby at the precise moment of birth or not.

Importantly, this wording leaves space for the mother to remain elevated as the one who truly "delivers" the baby. Using *midwife* as a verb encapsulates the complexity and dignity of a midwife's job during labor and birth in all its forms and manifestations. This is a creative way of using language to convey important truths about midwives at a time when there is great confusion in the general public over the differing roles of doulas, doctors, and nurses.

My friend Elizabeth Davis, a midwife, author, and speaker who teaches around the world, told me recently that she, too, has been talking for years about using the word *midwife* as a verb. She gave me this quote to share here that really sums it up:

> Midwifing may be practiced not only in terms of perinatal care, but in all aspects of life. We midwife when we bear witness, body and soul, to someone's pain, frustration, sadness, or grief. Midwifing can be done in any setting—in the corporate world at a challenging board meeting, in the supermarket line with someone having a meltdown, or in a difficult phone conversation with a customer service agent. In short, midwifery is a way of life!

Now let us turn our attention to a few mindsets our teams at Mercy In Action have cultivated over the years. Each one helps us do our work with greater skill and excellence. These ways of thinking guide us in our larger vision and strategy to strengthen the care we provide with intentionality.

MERCY IN ACTION'S "EXPECT THE UNEXPECTED" MINDSET

Before we can handle a birth emergency well, we must first prepare our minds. Understanding how the brain reacts in moments of crisis is one of the most valuable tools a midwife can have. When we understand what happens inside our own minds, we can learn to work with our brain instead of against it when every second matters.

Instinctive Denial Response

The human brain reacts in much the same way to any sudden life-threatening situation. Whether it is an earthquake, a car accident, or a birth that turns from calm to critical in an instant, our first thought is often "This cannot be happening." Even people who are well trained to work in crisis situations, such as paramedics and police officers, can experience that first moment of disbelief when something goes terribly wrong in front of their eyes. Denial can delay our response, and in birth work, delay can mean danger, as we know from the Three Delays model. The key to good outcomes is how fast we can break out of that initial denial that tends to freeze our thoughts and actions.

Researchers with the United States Department of Defense studied human reactions in fatal events and found something striking. In many cases, there was a brief window of time estimated at between five and seventy seconds, when a single action on the part of the victim could have changed the outcome and saved the person's life. This tells us that even in crisis, there is time to think, decide, and act, if we can do it quickly enough. For a midwife, that window of time may be the difference between a good outcome or a bad outcome for the mother, her baby, or both.

I will never forget the first time a laboring woman who had shown no previous warning signs suddenly went into a seizure. Her blood pressure had been normal throughout the labor. One minute she was chatting between her contractions, and the next her eyes rolled back as she collapsed into convulsions. My first thought was "This is not happening...there is no reason for this to be happening..."

The mind wants to protect itself from trauma by denying what it sees, and in those first crucial seconds when something terrible is coming down, our body often freezes as well. If we realize that this reaction is normal, we can overcome it. The key is to move quickly from denial to action. The faster we can unfreeze and accept what is happening, the greater the chance of survival, either for ourselves or for those we are responsible for keeping safe.

Awareness and Action

Awareness gives us power. We must retrain our minds to move quickly through disbelief and then act decisively to unfreeze our bodies within those first few seconds. Time is precious at the point of crisis, so preparation must begin in the mind long before the emergency begins in the room. Awareness is the first step toward survival in any crisis. It begins in the moment when your brain says, "This is not happening," and you deliberately and immediately answer back, "Yes, this is happening right now." That simple act of self-talk interrupts denial and brings the mind into the present.

Once awareness takes hold, the next step in a crisis is to make the decision to act. Begin by training yourself to move your body in some small, intentional way in response to fear. Physical movement breaks the paralysis that often comes with emotional shock. Even a simple motion, such as standing up, stepping forward, or reaching for supplies, tells the brain that it is time to respond, and that signal helps unlock the memory of what to do next so you can put together an appropriate action plan.

Kristen shared a relatable story with me while I was writing this chapter, telling me of the moment twenty years ago that she saw the umbilical cord swoosh out with the amniotic fluid during a labor she was attending. She said, "I distinctly remember my brain wanting to tell me I was not in fact seeing a cord." To override the denial, she moved her hand quickly to put on a sterile glove and lift the baby off the cord as she called loudly for others in the room to turn the mother and prepare for transport according to cord prolapse protocols. The story had a happy ending because she moved despite her instinctive denial and her previous training took over.

Since making an immediate decision is part of unfreezing, and there is not going to be time for ponderous thought, what will this decision be based on? The ability to make a quick plan of action and carry it out successfully depends on what is called "beforehand knowledge" and "survival capability." This includes the knowledge, training, and skills you already possess before the emergency begins, as well as the equipment, tools, and supplies you have available in your current environment. Together, these form the foundation on which your decisions are based, and the good news is, in most cases, you have some control over this part.

Beforehand Knowledge

Beforehand knowledge includes every bit of information in your brain on the subject, including the skills you possess. These skills fall into three categories: hand-eye coordination skills, also known as psychomotor skills, communication skills, and clinical decision-making skills. How useful all this will be to you in an emergent crisis depends on how much you have studied and practiced before the crisis occurs.

Prior real-life experience with a particular complication is not essential for the beforehand knowledge to be of use to you. For example, if a mother began to hemorrhage after birth, you would know from your midwifery education and training to act quickly to discern the cause and take action to stop the bleeding. You would know that most postpartum hemorrhages are caused by uterine atony, and you would know the steps to take and pharmacology to use to treat that condition. Your clinical decision-making skills would help you with the specifics, and you would use your communication skills to coordinate efforts among everyone in the room to ensure the mother's survival. Beforehand knowledge combines all your knowledge, learned skills and abilities, but it is most powerful when it is undergirded with strong muscle memory.

Muscle Memory

Muscle memory is what allows us to think clearly and respond without delay. To better understand what I mean by muscle memory, consider examples of performing complex motor skills such as playing a musical instrument, driving a car, or riding a bike. Things we do often, like tying our shoes or typing on a keyboard, become automatic through repetition. It's a neurological process where repeated practice allows the brain to perform movements more efficiently and with less conscious effort. So you can see how previous practice would be helpful before a crisis situation, and especially birth emergencies, since they are relatively rare.

Take a moment to think about your own skill set. Whether you are still learning the basics or are an experienced midwife, ask yourself if the foundational knowledge and abilities are already there in your brain to help you in any birth emergency. Do you refresh yourself on possible complications with regular reading and attending continuing education opportunities? Do you possess clinical skills such as suturing, IV insertion, resuscitation, and basic triage? And do you practice often enough to keep those skills sharp?

Awareness begins with knowing yourself and honestly assessing what you already carry in your mind and what you may need to strengthen. We control our beforehand knowledge, but this will only be a comfort to us if we have been diligent enough to keep learning and have committed to regularly reviewing emergency skills. If we do this, it is less likely that we will have to face a moment we are underprepared for. If there is a skill or complication you feel unsure about, now is the time to read up on it and practice it in simulation. Do not wait until you are called to a birth and find yourself wishing you had learned more about that one thing.

We once had a medical student who was very eager to learn and who was shadowing us at births. When a surprise breech baby was diagnosed one night, she told me that she had been hoping we would have a breech while she was with us. I looked at her and said, "So that means you studied up on breech delivery, then?" She looked sheepish and admitted that she had not.

American psychologist William James suggested that our experience will be what we agree to attend to. I told this medical student she would do well to study up on breech delivery and fill her mind with what to do before wishing for it, and that while most breech deliveries are uncomplicated, if a problem occurred and the head became stuck, there would not be time to look the solution up in a book.

The readiness that all birth workers need comes only by taking the time to study in advance and rehearse our skills until they become second nature. The families we serve have entrusted us with their safety, and they rightly expect us to be able to do whatever is necessary to help them safely through birth, normal or complicated. That is why we train, why we prepare, and why we plan our emergency supplies as if every item could make the difference between life and loss, because really, it could.

We have discussed the first two elements of being prepared to respond in a crisis. The first is awareness and action, accepting the situation and moving our bodies toward it. The second is beforehand knowledge, which is everything you already possess in your brain that allows you to take action, including your muscle memory. Now we turn our attention to the third and final piece: survival capability.

Survival Capability

Think of survival capability as the tools you have within reach to use in this emergency, and the ways your environment can help you and others survive the unplanned event. To picture this, imagine an earthquake has just occurred. You are on the third floor of a building that is now badly damaged, and a fire has broken out due to ruptured gas lines. The elevator does not work, and the stairs are blocked by fire. You look around and think, "What do I have here that could help me survive?" Maybe you pull the sheets and blankets off the bed, tie them securely together, and make a rope to lower yourself out the window. Maybe you see a fire-escape ladder out the window, but that window is painted shut, so you grab a cast-iron pan from the kitchen to smash out the window. Your ability to survive could also mean having a fully charged cell phone to call for help, or a flashlight to see in the dark. You make use of what is available to you in the moment as well as what has been prepared just in case. Now, bring that same idea of survival capacity into birth work.

At a moment's notice, we may be called upon to midwife a birth in a place we never expected. Ramona, one of our midwife school graduates in the 1990s, remembers when she was once summoned from our birth center in Davao by a husband asking for help getting his wife to the clinic, only to arrive at their tiny shack they called home to find the mother, pregnant with her ninth child, already pushing and unable to walk. With barely any space, she calmly asked for what little furniture they had to be moved around and created a clean birthing area within minutes. On another occasion, a laboring mother set out on foot for our birth center in Olongapo but made it no farther than a field along the path, and Ian was summoned to assist her where she lay. I have already told you about the extraordinary situation I found myself in when called upon to midwife a birth on an airplane, needing to adapt to the confined cabin space and nonexistent birth equipment. In each case—whether in a cramped shack, an open field, or at 30,000 feet—the midwife's work requires the ability to recognize when circumstances shift, to create order from chaos, and make use of whatever is available to function effectively when conditions are not ideal.

These moments reflect what we call survival capacity. It is the practiced readiness to respond with competence and calm in unpredictable environments, overcoming limitations and ensuring safety even when the setting or circumstances are unusually challenging.

At every birth, survival capability is largely dependent on what is available in the delivery room, or for a home birth, what you brought in your birth kit and what the family was required to prepare in advance. This means you should always ask yourself if you are truly prepared to meet the unexpected at the next birth you attend. Mercy In Action teaches a powerful continuing education course called Expect the Unexpected. To expect the unexpected, ask yourself questions like these: Is our equipment for any emergency in good working order? Are our medications current? Do we have a full oxygen tank, tubing, and the right size masks? Have we prepared adequately for anything that may occur?

In home birth kits, we recommend keeping everything needed for an IV insertion together including the solution, tubing, tape, alcohol pads, tourniquet, and IV catheter needles, ideally stored in a distinctive bag inside the main birth bag so that anyone could find it quickly without rummaging through pockets for separate pieces. In a birth center or hospital, drawers on the emergency crash cart should be clearly labeled so that nothing has to be searched for during an emergency while precious seconds slip away.

Survival capability also means making sure that everything you depend on is complete, current, and ready for use. A crisis is not the time to discover that a medicine has expired, a key item is missing, or a vital supply or tool was never replaced after the last use. Every birth bag, every cabinet, and every shelf in your birth center tells the story of your preparation, and your readiness can make all the difference when lives are at stake.

Some midwives have told me they prefer to leave emergency equipment in the car to avoid overwhelming the family at a home birth. I understand that instinct, but I always ask them to consider what would happen if the birth emergency response was needed immediately; who will go get the things from the car? Can your assistant find your car keys in a hurry, and do you really want to send your assistant away to get things when you may need her hands? What if it is night, or raining hard, or you parked far away? By the time someone runs outside and comes back, it may be too late for a timely response. Your equipment should be close enough to reach in seconds, not minutes. Also, an oxygen tank or IV fluids left in the car during cold weather could be unusable until it warms up. Some medications could be damaged from freezing or, conversely, from being left in a hot car in the summer.

The same principle of forward thinking applies to your physical setting. Many birth centers are converted homes; have you considered how easily a stretcher could fit through the doors or around corners in hallways if need be? Could emergency medical services reach every room quickly? If you attend home births, each house will present a new set of challenges. During prenatal visits, take time to evaluate each location. Can an ambulance easily find the home, or do numbers need to be painted on the house? I have known clients who wanted to give birth in their bed in a cozy cabin loft, but I ask them to imagine trying to carry the mother down the ladder on a stretcher in an emergency.

Preparation is what gives you control when everything else feels uncertain. You can't control the fact that unexpected complications will arise at times, but you do control your awareness, beforehand knowledge, and your survival capability. You get to determine what you put in your head and muscle memory. Most midwives have a say in what goes into your birth bag or is stocked on your crash cart. Preparation is everything when birth suddenly becomes complicated and life-defining decisions and actions need to be made. It is true in natural disasters as well as in birth: Controlling what you can control is essential for protecting and preserving life.

Making the Decision to Act

My sister worked in law enforcement for thirty years and specialized in crime prevention. Terri taught countless classes for women on self-defense, focusing on how to think clearly in dangerous situations and how to be prepared in advance for the best reaction if threatened. She generously taught personal safety to our midwives for years in workshops she created for Mercy In Action. Because of her work, she developed her own safety habits for traveling alone and staying in a hotel overnight. One was a simple alarm device that triggered a piercing sound if anyone tried to open the hotel door. On a business trip one night, she was awakened by the sound of her alarm device going off, alerting her that someone was opening her hotel room door in the middle of the night. She told me later that even with all her training, her first thought was, "This must be a mistake, the alarm must be malfunctioning." Her brain at first refused to accept that the danger was real. But because she had been so well trained to recognize the trick her brain was playing, she took action and immediately leapt out of bed in the dark room, yelling toward the door at the top of her lungs, "Get out of here!"

She had made a plan in advance for this kind of situation should it ever happen, and had practiced it, and that muscle memory took over as she made her voice loud, angry, and commanding. It worked; she heard the intruder's footsteps running down the hall. That story stayed with me. The lessons are there in this story: Even if we are experienced, the brain will try to trick us, but we can overcome that handicap by being aware of this reaction, having a prearranged plan, and moving our body (and our voice) to put the plan into action.

When a newborn emerges not breathing, I have seen an inexperienced midwife keep rubbing the baby longer than they should before moving to the next step of giving ventilation breaths. We get stuck because it has usually worked before to rub the baby, and our minds take a while to process the situation and accept that it is not working this time.

Denial keeps us frozen, whereas making a decision activates the brain to unfreeze. However, you must have decided ahead of time what you will do, and you must remember how to do it. That is why we practice our drills. You cannot use what you do not have, and you cannot remember what you never learned. Preparation must happen long before the emergency.

A successful response to a birth complication or emergency is a combination of training, experience, judgment, and practice. Role-playing is the best type of ongoing practice there is, because it builds muscle memory, those neural pathways that memory lays down through repetition. When we practice a skill repeatedly, the brain builds a route that allows us to respond automatically on the day we need to use it in real life. In a crisis, those practiced responses can override fear and hesitation, allowing us to jump into action when every second matters.

Our job as midwives is to protect the normal when everything goes well, and to protect life when things shift unexpectedly and a dangerous deviation from normal occurs.

MERCY IN ACTION'S PERSON OVERBOARD DRILLS

I mentioned in the previous chapter that I gained a key insight from my time touring a ship in our local harbor. There was a second take-away that came to me while talking to the ship's captain that day, an insight that inspired our Person Overboard Drills, which we use to this day in all our birth centers.

The MV Logos Hope, known at the time as the world's largest floating bookstore, entered our harbor in Subic Bay, the Philippines, in the spring of 2012. Mercy In Action was honored when our local leadership team received an invitation to have a special tour of the ship. You should know that this ship was crewed by young volunteers from fifty-six different nations who lived and worked on board. As I was being given a tour by the captain, I wondered how they managed communication with so many different languages spoken.

I noticed the life rafts strapped to the side and asked the captain how they prepared for the possibility of someone falling overboard. He explained that they practiced emergency drills every single week, a full drill that included unroping and dropping the life rafts into the sea. Curious, I asked how often someone fell overboard. His answer surprised me—he said it had never happened yet. I asked how long they had been sailing, and he said fourteen years. I had to stop him and make sure I understood. "Wait," I said, "you mean you practice person overboard drills every single week for fourteen years in anticipation of an emergency event that has happened exactly never?" He nodded and said, "That is right."

In that moment, I realized what we often miss in midwifery. Consistent practice for birth emergencies is not required after we graduate from midwifery school, with the exception of recertification in adult and newborn resuscitation. While we learn about all the possible complications during preservice training, we could let years go by without thinking about the rare ones that happen only once in a great while.

I have overheard midwives' reasoning that rare complications are not worth focusing on. While teaching workshops on shock and IV therapy over the years, I have been told by more than one participant that they used to carry certain emergency drugs or supplies, but they never had to use it before the expiration date, so they did not think it worthwhile to replace their stock.

Midwifery that is strategic and service-oriented is not only about being present for what is normal and routine but also about preparing for the unexpected. True readiness means planning ahead for the events we hope will never happen. The fact is, birth complications are rare in a low-risk population, and even in a high-risk population, most women will birth normally, and babies will come out and breathe on their own. But to train diligently and rehearse for those rare instances, so that no one dies of a preventable cause, seems not only reasonable but ethical and essential to good maternity care.

Repetition builds readiness. In instigating the concept of our Person Overboard Drills, we are saying we want to be like that ship's captain.

Someday, it might happen that a person falls overboard on the Logos Hope, and on that day, it is highly likely that person will be rescued and survive. The crew has practiced so many times that their response is second nature, and every detail has already been worked out in advance. Wouldn't it be good if the same could be true for rare and dangerous birth emergencies? Imagine your relief when the unthinkable happens, but no one dies from a preventable cause, because you were diligent in practicing those skills over the years, never knowing when they may be needed. I always remember that the ship captain did not say people don't fall overboard; he said on his ship it had not happened "yet..."

Hard Lessons

Observing the ship's protocols was my personal tipping point, after previously hearing my sister's stories and taking classes in disaster response and wilderness first aid. When I returned to our birth center after touring the ship, I told our midwife staff we were going to start scheduling regular birth complication and emergency practice drills.

The timing could not have been more sobering. Only weeks earlier, our midwife team had lost a baby during a rare but serious complication where the baby's umbilical cord had prolapsed out of the mother's vagina before birth, which basically cuts off oxygen. The midwife in charge that day knew the skills to perform and responded correctly at first, placing the mother in the knee-chest position and holding the head off the cord with her gloved hand. Unfortunately, we had never practiced communicating under pressure with emergency personnel. When the ambulance arrived, the uniformed men took over, and the midwife, unsure how to assert herself in this situation, did as they commanded and stepped back. The pregnant mother was placed flat on her back in the ambulance, and by the time they reached the hospital, her baby was gone.

It was a painful loss, full of remorse and recrimination, and it reminded us that skill alone is not enough. What made it even harder was that ten years earlier, we had faced the same complication with a very different outcome. Back then, our team was working in a small mountain town in the northern Philippines, and one day a cord prolapse occurred during labor. The midwives moved quickly. They carried the mother to our vehicle in the correct position, with the attending midwife's hand remaining inside to lift the baby's head and protect the cord all the way to the hospital.

When they arrived at the tiny provincial hospital, there were no doctors on duty. Our midwife refused to lower her hand even when told to do so by the confused nursing staff who had never seen this procedure, because she knew what was at stake. Her husband realized how urgent the situation was and drove off to find the surgeon at his home and the anesthesiologist at the nearby church attending mass, and drove them both back to the hospital. After all that delay, against all odds, the baby was delivered by cesarean with good Apgar scores. A life was saved that day.

Those two cord prolapse events happened ten years apart; juxtaposed, they showed that even with the same emergency, the outcome depends on how ready we are, not just in skill, but in confidence and communication. We now regularly rehearse every part of a birth emergency, from hands-on response to the words we use when others enter the room, including practicing the telephone call we make for referral.

Objective Structured Clinical Evaluation

We use OSCEs for these examinations (Objective Structured Clinical Examinations, although in our organization we refer to them as Objective Structured Clinical Evaluations). If you have ever taken a CPR or NRP course, you are already familiar with the concept of an OSCE. An OSCE simply provides a checklist to guide you through each step of a scenario, making sure nothing is missed. But the real strength of these drills lies in the teamwork, communication, and confidence that grow through practice. We rehearse as if it were real, down to the last detail: how to recognize an emergency, how to move quickly to begin our medical response, how to coordinate a safe transfer to a hospital if needed, and what to say on the phone to emergency medical personnel. Throughout the pretend scenario, we practice how to stay calm and clear minded. Mercy In Action's OSCEs have become a vital part of our training in every birth center, helping us feel confident rather than fearful because we know exactly what to do if the unthinkable occurs. When the real emergency comes, we want to be like that ship's crew, ready for the day someone falls overboard, ready to rescue them without a hitch.

Now, let us turn to a different kind of mindset, one that keeps us steady and clear when birth is unfolding normally. It may seem the opposite of preparing for emergencies, but actually both are on the same spectrum of readiness, grounded in respect for birth and responsibility for life.

MERCY IN ACTION'S SAFE LABOR SPECTRUM

Mercy In Action's Safe Labor Spectrum concept keeps us keenly focused on the situation at any given moment and on our appropriate role in the response. It is a deliberate and conscious choice to stay acutely aware of what is unfolding. I developed this concept to help midwives tailor their approach, being continually aware of the spectrum of possibilities present at every labor.

We can trust birth because it is a normal physiological function of the human reproductive system. In the same way that other systems of the body are designed to work efficiently and without help on our part, such as the respiratory and digestive systems, the reproductive system is remarkably capable and finely tuned to sustain pregnancy, bring forth new life, and establish breastfeeding. Our task as midwives is to guard these natural processes of the body by avoiding unnecessary disruptions and unhelpful meddling.

However, no system in the body is without flaw. The lungs may falter with asthma or pneumonia and need help to get back to normal. The digestive tract may struggle with heartburn or ulcers and require medications. Bones can break and hearts can require surgery. Similarly, the reproductive system, although usually dependable, can sometimes present unexpected complications, whether minor or severe. For midwives to recognize the moment we are in, and whether the situation calls upon us to do nothing or to do everything, is essential for achieving the best birth outcomes.

The philosophy of midwifery care that I have personally developed and taught my midwife teams to use over decades of practice rests on a simple but critical principle: Do nothing to help or do everything to help, but stay out of the muddy middle. Don't fiddle when labor is working, and don't dawdle if labor becomes dangerous to the mother or baby.

The midwife's role is to watch carefully and respond appropriately, keeping both mother and baby within the safest possible passage. The Safe Labor Spectrum helps by reminding us to continually evaluate the labor's status at any given moment. If labor is working just fine, then talking or suggesting some change only disrupts the natural process. Birth attendants can likewise make the mistake of assuming labor will always be straightforward. I have seen midwives unconsciously assume a doula role, all comfort and no vital sign monitoring, during an intense and painful birth. This is how devastating complications such as uterine rupture can be missed until too late.

Our goal in every labor is to avoid the tragedy of too little too late or too much too soon. Remember that the goal is "just right" maternity care. Any intervention should be the right amount at the right time in the right way.

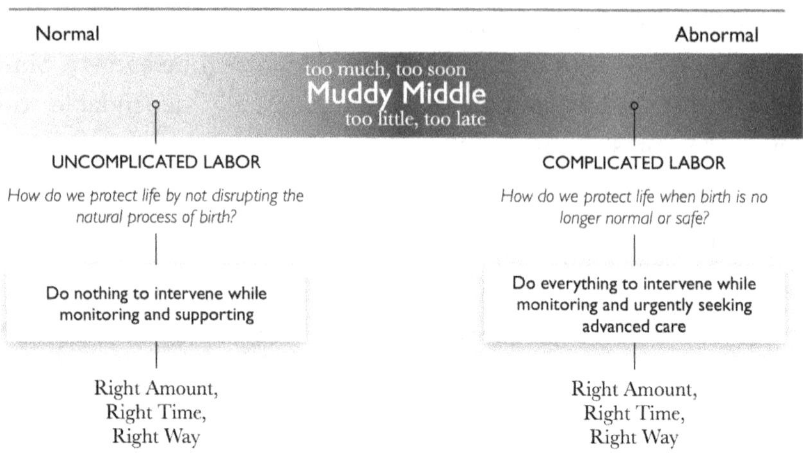

The labor spectrum concept reminds us that we cannot improve on a process that is already working; to try is to disrupt it. We want to stay as far to the left side of the spectrum as possible when birth is working. Likewise, we want to avoid the deadly delays and recognize a problem quickly. If a complication arises, we want to quickly move to the right side of the spectrum, now offering the help and intervention that will make labor survivable for the mother and baby.

Smart Midwifery

Smart midwifery is a term I have coined to describe the astute midwife's way of being. Smart midwifery means using all your senses to observe while doing nothing to help when birth is working, using all your skills to do everything needed to help when birth becomes life-threatening, and honing the astute ability to always know the difference.

Smart midwifery is the art of discernment. It requires skill and diligence to constantly evaluate for risk factors without disturbing the natural process of birth. It is not easy to have the discipline and self-control to refrain from unnecessary "helping" when birth is working on its own. When birth is progressing smoothly, unfolding just as it should, even well-meaning comfort measures given at the wrong time in the wrong way can disrupt the process and trigger a complication.

Smart midwifery during a normal birth is hands-off, watchful, and respectful; this is the ideal way to keep both the mother and baby safe. Yet the midwife must remain vigilant, taking and recording vital signs often throughout labor to confirm that all continues to be normal with both the mother and her baby, first inside and later outside of the womb. At the other end of the spectrum lies the possibility that complications may emerge slowly over time or strike at a moment's notice. In those situations, midwives must be ready to act swiftly and decisively, using every skill available to safeguard life. Smart midwifery is not about halfway measures; it is about knowing when to stand back completely and when to move in and use every skill and resource at your disposal.

If the birth attendant interferes when birth is working, they risk creating a cascade of complications with further interventions becoming necessary, all of which can cause harm. If the birth attendant fails to intervene promptly and decisively when complications arise, harm may come to the mother, baby, or both as a result. This is why midwifery wisdom calls us to stay out of the muddy middle and instead commit ourselves to one side of the labor spectrum or the other, using discernment that protects both mother and child during both straightforward labors and those labors that become complicated.

The Dutch Hallway

In 1987, I was introduced by Dr. Michel Odent to a Dutch midwife, Beatrijs Smulders, and we quickly bonded as friends and colleagues. Beatrijs invited me to attend a home birth with her in Amsterdam, and she later visited me in Alaska and attended a birth in my birth center. Our ways were very much aligned, as we both held deep convictions about not disrupting normal birth, but she showed me how to be even more hands off and trusting of the process.

While I was in the Netherlands, Beatrijs made it possible for me to visit a teaching hospital where midwives were being trained under the guidance of the illustrious obstetrician G. J. Kloosterman. He had recently given a famous talk, remembered as the "five minutes to midnight" speech, in which he warned that Dutch midwifery stood at a crossroads; the system could either follow the global drift toward highly medicalized birth, or it could preserve its unique and very successful model of independent, autonomous midwifery with home birth at its core.

The Dutch had already proven the value of their model, with some of the best maternal and newborn outcomes in the world, and they had retained traditional home birth into their national system in a way that was getting excellent outcomes. Beatrijs was one of the midwives on the front lines of pulling the country back from its slide toward medicalized birth. During my time with her, I learned a lot about the model of maternity care in the Netherlands. One of the things that struck me most was the way they trained their midwives.

In the Dutch system, all midwives were taught to think like home birth midwives, even those practicing in hospitals. Everyone was trained to start from the assumption that birth is normal. Midwives were primarily trained in a teaching hospital setting, which is common for midwife training in much of the world. However, the Dutch system was strikingly different in that if a complication arose, the midwife did not simply summon a doctor to the room. Instead, the birthing mother was transferred across the hall, from the normal birth side to the medical side. This practice created a clear boundary in thinking: As long as labor was progressing normally, care remained on one side of the hall, in the hands of midwives. If a situation shifted to high-risk, then the woman is transported across the corridor, where medical staff joined the midwife collaboratively to provide the necessary interventions needed to keep the birth safe.

Doctors and midwives respect each other, and everyone works together for the common goal of supporting patients during childbirth.

Observing this with my own eyes made a deep impression on me. It was such a tangible reminder that the way we structure systems can either cloud or clarify our judgment. The system in the Netherlands had found a way to protect normal birth while ensuring safety in emergencies. Even today, with home birth rates in the Netherlands higher than any other high-income country, the wisdom of that model continues to stand out to me and serves as a clear example of smart midwifery using a form of my safe labor spectrum concept.

Recognizing Normal

When I am mentoring students, and they tell me a particular labor is normal, I ask them, "How do you know this labor is normal?" The only real way to know that birth is progressing normally is through frequent monitoring of vital signs, careful and detailed observation, and attentive listening to the mother, both her words and unspoken body language.

A good midwife practices observation much the same way the fictional character Sherlock Holmes did, with precise attention, disciplined perception, and an almost scientific habit of noticing. This kind of seeing is guided by curiosity and meticulous attention to detail, tuning in to slight shifts and catching subtle clues that reveal whether birth is progressing normally or when something is beginning to change for the worse. It is a practice of observation leading to careful deduction.

To do this well, we must be aware of all the ways that we can be distracted. For instance, knitting or crocheting at a birth can be a good activity for staying calm and centered in between vital sign checks at a long labor, but only if you are already a master knitter and don't need to concentrate on technique or count stitches. Reading a book, on the other hand, is never a good idea, as books transport us to another place and time, and we can easily get lost in them. The same is true for smartphones; they are attention stealers and wildly distracting, making it easy to lose track of time and space while scrolling. So, unless you are briefly looking something up, stay away from books, and except when you are doing electronic records charting, stay away from screens during labor watches.

The Safe Labor Spectrum is a way of picturing the range between doing "too much too soon" and "too little too late," and noting that the target is to provide maternity care that is "the right amount at the right time in the right way." Let's take a moment to be clear on why many routine practices during labor that may seem innocuous can be harmful to the natural process of birth.

The Brain in Labor

Let's unpack the science of why interventions, big or small, during a normal labor can be harmful. Labor begins and progresses because of hormones, and something extraordinary takes place in the human brain under their influence, so it is helpful to know a bit about how this works. In simple terms, the neocortex—the thinking part of the brain that plans, analyzes, and solves problems—quietly steps aside while the limbic brain takes over. The limbic brain is the instinctive center of emotion, memory, and primal function, and it takes the lead once labor reaches an advanced state. This shift allows birth to unfold physiologically. With the limbic brain in charge, oxytocin is released in steady pulses, contractions eventually grow stronger and closer together, endorphins are released to ease the pain, and the groundwork is laid for immediate bonding and the start of breastfeeding at the moment of birth.

This delicate balance, however, can be easily disrupted. Pain medication throws it off, and so does talking to the mother or any disturbance caused by well-meaning helpers at the birth. The neocortex is quick to reawaken with conversation, bright lights, distracting noises, or the feeling of being observed. When that happens, adrenaline rises, hormone activity may slow, and labor can stall. That is why once hard labor begins, it is crucial not to interrupt with unnecessary chatter or efforts to be overly helpful. Adrenaline is the enemy of oxytocin, the hormone necessary for birth to occur naturally.

Even suggesting a position change or telling a mother to push (in the absence of a problem) is now recognized as unhelpful interference in her ability to listen to her own body and give birth instinctively. The International Childbirth Initiative lists caregiver-directed pushing on a prohibited list of non-evidence-based actions during normal labor, as research has found it to be an unnatural and unhelpful intervention. Birth is safest when the mother feels private, safe, and supported, free to sink into that altered state often dubbed as "labor land," where her limbic brain can guide the work her body was designed to do. If she can remain undisturbed in this state as she enters second stage, she may experience the fetal ejection reflex, a powerful, involuntary physiological response that causes the baby to be born rapidly with minimal effort. This is the safest kind of birth for both mother and baby.

It cannot be overemphasized that only close monitoring gives us the confidence to do nothing in a normal labor, and only close monitoring allows us to recognize an unfolding complication before it becomes life threatening. The baby in the womb cannot tell you if they feel distress; you must listen carefully to the count and rhythm of the fetal heartbeat. In the same way, a mother's blood pressure and pulse are invisible until measured. This is why taking vital signs at frequent intervals is essential and must never be delayed or neglected. It can definitely be done in a way that does not disturb the natural flow of labor hormones. I am very good at quietly and unobtrusively getting vital signs in labor; it is a skill I have perfected over time.

Abiding by the Safe Labor Spectrum means that, whether the birth is entirely normal or a complication occurs at some point, the right response will be obvious, and the midwife will be able to act accordingly. Cross the metaphorical hall quickly and completely when necessary—never halfway, never dithering in the in-between places. Stay on one side or the other, and be deeply cognizant of when, how, and why you might choose to interfere. The goal is to interfere only with complications but never with the normal process of labor.

MINDSET MATTERS

Staying cognizant of how to provide maternity care that is just right, neither over-interventive nor underprepared, is not simply a practice; it is a mindset. It calls us to stay fully conscious of our presence in the birth space, to be careful never to disturb the instinctual rhythm of labor, while remaining ready to act with clarity and precision when the unexpected occurs. To be both calm and decisive, trusting in nature while staying vigilant and always being prepared for anything, is the essence of skilled midwifery. Midwifery at its best is both science and art. We practice, we plan, we strategize, because every mother deserves safety, every baby deserves a fair start, and every birth worker deserves the peace of mind of knowing we are ready to do our job well when it matters most.

In the next chapter, we will take a deep dive into another visionary strategy that Mercy In Action uses to extend our reach and change lifelong outcomes for the babies in our care: our First 1,000 Days program.

PAUSE FOR REFLECTION

What practices do you use to keep normal labor undisturbed while still monitoring vital signs frequently? In what ways do you prepare with your birth team to be ready for the next birth emergency? What habits can you put in place to make emergency drills a routine practice in your setting?

8
SHAPING A STRONG START

Children are not the people of tomorrow, but are people of today.

— JANUSZ KORCZAK

One of the universal joys of midwifery is running into a client or patient months or even years after the birth and seeing them with the child you helped welcome into the world. I began my midwifery journey back in 1980, so I've had the privilege of many reconnections with families whose babies are now grown. I have met children of the children I once midwifed, and now it's even to the third generation, as I meet their grandchildren! There's a quiet pride many of us have as we see "our babies" growing up in the community.

The impetus for our Mercy In Action First 1,000 Days program in our Philippine birth centers was an encounter I had while walking down the road with one of our Filipina midwives. On this particular day, a woman approached us, and I was delighted to recognize one of our postpartum mothers, Carmen. She had delivered a baby at our birth center the year before. As we greeted her and asked how the family was, she told us through tears that her one-year-old baby had recently gotten sick, gone downhill rapidly, and died the month before. Carmen gave us this tragic news in a voice full of sadness and apparent resignation. We hugged her and offered our sympathy and a prayer right there on the street. As we walked away, my midwife friend said, "It happens here." A heaviness settled over me, because I knew childhood deaths were all too common in the impoverished areas our birth centers serve. I had already witnessed more of them than I felt my heart could bear in one lifetime.

Carmen had answered "diarrhea" when I asked what happened, but the cause could just as well have been pneumonia, measles, or any one of the common childhood illnesses that prey on the young. The story was all too familiar to me. A baby leaves our birth center in good health in the arms of smiling parents, only to die needlessly in early childhood. We may have accompanied the mother safely through a high-risk pregnancy or managed a harrowing delivery; we may have saved the baby's life through resuscitation after birth; but despite our best efforts to give this child a good start in life, he has a significant chance of dying young from a disease of deprivation.

The tragedy of these preventable deaths is an overwhelming global problem, seemingly too big to make a dent in. Child deaths often share a comorbidity with chronic malnutrition, a risk that stalks babies when their mother weans them from the breast. After we met Carmen on the road, I started pondering how we could at least set up a safety net in our own context. I was heartbroken, tired of feeling helpless, and aching to break out of the paralyzing sense of fatalism that is so pervasive in poor communities. I began to dream of the day our entire team would see early childhood deaths as a problem that requires our intervention, not a hopeless inevitability for far too many of our babies after they leave our care.

SURVIVE AND THRIVE

Even in high-mortality areas, midwives with vision and purpose should not be satisfied with our patients simply surviving until they leave our care at six weeks postpartum. We want them to live long and thrive, in all aspects of their lives. That is my hope and prayer for each and every little one in our care, no matter the circumstances the parents are facing. Although the statistics we keep are important, if we measure success only by survival rates, we are missing something vital. Survival is the floor, the bare minimum. Thriving is the ceiling, and that is what we must truly be reaching for when we get involved in maternity care.

Survival is life, but thriving is life more abundant. One key to seeing a vision of life more abundant come true for every one of our babies is to focus on the most vulnerable time in a person's life—their first 1,000 days, described as the time in the womb up to the second birthday.

In this chapter you will find another secret to success in Mercy In Action's intentional healthcare delivery model that goes beyond pregnancy and birth into early childhood, with creativity and a focus on the future.

WHAT CAN MIDWIVES DO?

In Mercy In Action's ministry, our birth centers are midwife-led, meaning the midwives not only attend to pregnant women and their babies but also have the greatest potential to influence the parents' attitudes and behaviors during pregnancy and beyond.

Although professional midwives are responsible for the care of babies, both in the womb and for six weeks after birth, few midwives I have spoken with understand the role that the first 1,000 days of life play in a child's health and well-being. If midwives can facilitate parents learning about this, it could improve long-term survival and protect the child's health and future ability to thrive in school, work, and life. Midwives have a unique opportunity to help shape destinies and unlock potentials far beyond childhood by using the educational opportunities present during pregnancy.

Reading the book *The First 1,000 Days* solidified my understanding of this critical phase in a child's life. Written by Roger Thurow, a journalist with an extensive background in researching world hunger, the book details the importance of the first 1,000 days of a child's life by focusing on nutrition, hygiene, healthcare, and parental love and attention. The author follows pregnant women in four countries where the odds are stacked against raising healthy children due to poverty, discrimination, and the lack of resources.

In places such as my adopted home, the Philippines, effective maternal and child health strategies often depend on strong partnerships between governments and nongovernmental organizations (NGOs), since public health funding alone cannot meet the full scope of need. Nonprofit mission and charity NGOs like Mercy In Action are often invited to stand in the gap, offering care, education, and support that strengthen families and improve outcomes across generations. This shared focus is built on collaboration, and it is in that spirit of global solidarity and shared concern for children that we launched our First 1,000 Days program in our birth centers in the Philippines, which I will describe in this chapter.

I want to make clear, though, that the First 1,000 Days is a universal concept that is needed everywhere, in both rich and poor countries. All midwives and birth workers, including doulas and childbirth educators, should thoroughly understand how to explain the importance of this timeframe to parents during pregnancy, as it is a powerful tool that can significantly impact a child's health throughout their lifetime. With that in mind, we launched an online continuing education course years ago called Midwives & The First 1,000 Days that focuses on both high and low-income settings.

It is an extraordinary truth that the future of entire nations is shaped by the quality of nutrition and loving interaction during the first 1,000 days of a child's life, when most brain cells are formed and vital connections within the brain are made. Childhood malnutrition has been called a silent emergency because the damage it causes can be difficult to see, yet its effects last a lifetime. The same is true of neglect and lack of stimulation. Midwives are uniquely positioned to help prevent this hidden harm by teaching families the importance of the entire first 1,000 days, not just pregnancy and birth.

At Mercy In Action, we see our role now as undergirding parents in a way that makes the First 1,000 Days a tangible guide for action. But before I tell you about how our program integrates midwifery, early childhood development, and public health, let me explain why this concept is so important for the survival and thriving of children everywhere that babies are being born.

1,000 DAYS TIMEFRAME

The first 1,000 days of life are defined as beginning at conception and culminating at the child's second birthday. Breaking it down into phases, the first phase spans the nine months of pregnancy. The second phase is infancy, further broken into two parts for a breastfeeding baby—the six months of exclusive breastfeeding, and the next six months of breastfeeding along with solid food introduction. The third and final phase is called early childhood, stretching from one year old to two years old, a time of transition to the family diet.

CHAMPIONING A FAIR START

The first 1,000 days are a window of opportunity to enable each child to reach their potential. When I teach this to midwives and birth workers, I often use the metaphor of a race to understand the concept of a fair start. What if a foot race is set to begin, with some children already standing at the starting line, while others start so far back that they can never catch up?

Every child deserves the opportunity to reach the potential that was woven into their being from the moment of conception. Yet millions of children are born without that chance, because it is robbed from them in the womb or shortly after. They may live in unstable or unsafe environments, lack the food their growing bodies need, or have parents who simply do not know how to provide the proper nutrition and stimulation that their children require. Poverty, hunger, and lack of education create barriers that hold children back before they even begin. When that happens, a child starts life at a disadvantage, one that may begin in the womb and carry forward into every stage of development.

Researchers have found that early setbacks in life can make it harder to get an education, find good work, and live a healthy life. It may even affect the ability to maintain healthy relationships. Many experts now believe this is one of the root causes of the inequality and generational poverty that persist across societies. Improving a child's first 1,000 days will not solve every problem, but it offers a powerful opportunity to interrupt that cycle and build more equitable beginnings. Then children can start the race of life side by side, rather than too many being left behind.

Evidence shows that children have the best chance for a healthy future when they benefit from the following: early prenatal care and good nutrition in the womb, a safe and gentle birth, early and exclusive breastfeeding followed by nutritious table food started at six months, mental and emotional nurturing, play and exercise, and protection from disease. When every child is given the chance to thrive, everyone benefits. Midwives have a vital role in this transformation. We stand at the beginning of life, where the trajectory of health and hope has the potential to impact generations and entire nations.

As midwives know, the well-being of a child is intertwined with that of their mother right from the start. Yet access to prenatal care remains unequal in many parts of the world. Some women cannot afford care; others may be eligible for government programs but cannot enroll without first being seen by a doctor, creating a delay in starting care if appointments are backed up or money to pay is lacking. In some communities, women live too far from a prenatal clinic or are too busy working to put food on the table to attend regular appointments. There are countless barriers that prevent women from receiving care when it matters most.

Researchers now suggest that inequalities in child development often begin before birth. Poverty, food insecurity, and limited prenatal care affect both the mother's health and that of her growing baby. Even in wealthy countries, pregnant women may live in food deserts where fresh, healthy food is out of reach, and more and more rural hospitals are closing their maternity units, forcing pregnant women to drive for hours to access prenatal care.

While even mild food deprivation during pregnancy can have lasting negative effects, and we know prenatal care is a crucial element of a healthy pregnancy, stress is another hidden factor. Depression and anxiety, which elevate stress hormones during pregnancy, can affect a baby's development in the womb, leading to cognitive delays, attention difficulties, and emotional challenges later in life. Of course, when we talk about this to pregnant women, we must be careful not to increase their stress. Instead, our aim is to identify and relieve it. As midwives, we seek to lighten burdens, foster stability, and support peaceful, healthy pregnancies whenever possible.

Midwives and pediatricians all over the world know that breastfeeding provides the best brain-building benefits and gives babies the healthiest start in life. This is true in the physical, emotional, and social realm. Yet too many women lack the support they need to begin or to continue breastfeeding. It is common knowledge that unscrupulous formula company reps pay midwives and doctors to peddle their artificial milk products, sabotaging breastfeeding. Low-income mothers and those in marginalized communities often face greater challenges. Cultural attitudes and limited workplace accommodations can interfere. Many women do not have jobs that allow time to nurse or pump, and in many countries, there is still no paid maternity leave or workplace protection for breastfeeding mothers.

How long a mother breastfeeds her baby often correlates with her income and education. Wealthier and more educated women tend to breastfeed longer, while others face barriers that make it difficult to sustain. If we truly want every baby to have a fair start, we must pay special attention to those mothers who fall outside the circle of privilege, and ensure they receive the support and encouragement they need to succeed.

SAFEGUARDING THE CHILD'S BRAIN

Good nutrition during the first 1,000 days provides the building blocks for healthy brain development, starting with good nutrition during pregnancy, and the start of breastfeeding within the first hour of birth. This is something midwives should already understand, and we could extend our impact by using this phrase and explaining the concept of the First 1,000 Days when we discuss food and breastfeeding with parents. We could extensively discuss the power of breastfeeding for the growing brain and encourage continued breastfeeding throughout the first year at least. Although in many settings midwifery care concludes at six weeks after the birth, there are things we can stress in our prenatal education and postpartum advice that will stick with the parents long after they officially leave our maternity care.

During prenatal education, we can teach parents and extended family members how essential playing, reading, and positive stimulation are for their baby's brain growth. Simple acts of holding, cuddling, and carrying a baby close strengthen neural connections and emotional security. From the first moments after birth and throughout early childhood, these everyday gestures of love help build a healthy, responsive brain.

There are so many advantages of early prenatal care that we need to be creative in thinking up ways to provide it. Perhaps offering clinic hours that match working women's schedules, conducting outreach, or organizing group prenatal visits around childbirth education and parenting gatherings are some ideas to try. Ideally, we should also be offering pre-pregnancy and early pregnancy classes in our communities. That is what I did in Alaska; several times a year, we advertised a free class in the community called How to Grow a Healthy Baby, which was always well attended.

For the safest and best first 1,000 days, we should never ask pregnant women to wait to begin prenatal care. Some providers are in the habit of waiting to schedule the first visit until the end of the first trimester, but once we understand the significance of the first 1,000 days, we realize how essential it is to begin as early as possible. Early counseling on good nutrition and the avoidance of teratogens (substances and environmental factors that can harm a developing fetus) helps every baby get the healthiest possible start.

BRAIN DEVELOPMENT IN PREGNANCY

The child's time in the womb begins the process of building the brain that will shape their future cognitive abilities, motor skills, and emotional development. Nutrition and environment during pregnancy set the foundation for learning and health long before birth. These early months and years form a powerful window of growth, influencing how a child will learn, thrive in school, and even succeed economically later in life.

The opposite is also true. A child's rapidly developing brain is especially vulnerable to neglect, either from poor nutrition or lack of attention. There is also a toxic kind of stress that accompanies a pregnancy marked by hunger, depression, or domestic violence. Babies in the womb experience deprivations too, sensing if the mother is in distress from food insecurity or an unsafe environment.

Early brain development is an area where midwives have tremendous influence to shape a better future for at-risk children. There are many ways we can protect and strengthen this critical period of growth. A child's brain begins to grow very early in pregnancy, and it develops at an astonishing speed. By the fourth week, the brain already contains thousands of cells, and by the twenty-fourth week, it contains billions. In just twenty weeks in the womb, the transformation is extraordinary. The nutrition a baby receives from the mother's diet is the fuel that drives this rapid brain growth.

Nutrients such as folic acid, iron, zinc, iodine, protein, and fatty acids all play essential roles in the development of the baby's brain during pregnancy. When one or more of these nutrients are lacking, the baby may face developmental delays or even birth defects that can result in permanent cognitive challenges. Because the mother's diet and nutrient stores are the baby's only source of nourishment, it is vital that midwives teach expectant mothers how to eat a healthy diet and help them access nutritious food. We can encourage support systems that make healthy choices possible and address food insecurity. We can screen for depression and be aware of the signs of domestic violence. Our job should be to remove barriers whenever possible so that every baby gets the best start possible.

BRAIN DEVELOPMENT IN INFANCY

The building of a baby's brain does not stop at birth. During infancy, the brain continues to grow at an incredible pace. Breast milk supports not only physical health but also brain development. It is nature's perfect food, rich in nutrients, proteins, growth factors, and hormones that cannot be replicated in a formula. It is personalized nourishment, changing as the baby grows, uniquely created for each baby's stage of development. Breastfed babies have been shown to have higher IQs.

Breastfeeding also strengthens the emotional connection between mother and child. The distance between the mother's eyes and the baby at the breast is exactly the range at which newborns can focus best, allowing for deep bonding through eye contact. The touch and closeness during breastfeeding build the baby's sensory and emotional pathways in the brain, which are essential for later cognitive and emotional development.

If, for some reason, breastfeeding is not possible, expressed milk from the baby's own mother is next best, followed by donor milk when available. If formula feeding is necessary, everything is more challenging, but feeding should still be a nurturing experience, with the baby held close and fed in a way that mirrors the emotional warmth of breastfeeding. These acts of connection and care fuel both body and brain, forming the foundation for healthy growth throughout the first 1,000 days.

One of the most heartbreaking things I have seen working in low-resource communities is the sight of skinny babies with a worried expression on their faces. It is striking because babies are not supposed to look distressed. These malnourished babies may end up this way due to artificial milk feeding with unhygienic bottles, unclean water sources, and watered-down powdered milk not meant for a baby. Even in infancy, babies can experience the stress of hunger and food insecurity, which harms both their developing brains and their overall health. The damage caused by poor nutrition during the earliest days, beginning in pregnancy and continuing after birth, can be profound and often irreversible.

BRAIN DEVELOPMENT IN EARLY CHILDHOOD

Now let's turn to the next stage of development, early childhood. I realize this is often beyond the direct scope of midwifery practice, but it remains an important time for us to influence through our counsel and encouragement. While mothers and babies are still in our care, we can help lay a strong foundation that will carry over into these next formative years.

Small children need big nutrition to fuel their growing brains and prepare them for learning. Toddlerhood is a season of amazing growth, and young children need to eat several times a day to get enough calories since their stomachs are small. As a baby moves into this stage, the brain continues to develop at a remarkable pace. By age two, a child's brain has reached about 80% of its adult size. During the first year alone, it doubles in size, and structural changes, such as the expansion of white matter and rapid synapse formation, continue throughout the second year.

During early childhood, the brain is busy forming trillions of connections, building the networks that shape thinking, memory, and language. Even before a child can speak, they are already learning language. Every sound, facial expression, and word they hear is helping to build the architecture of communication. Loving care helps babies form brain connections that wire them to trust that the world is safe. In contrast, exposure to violence, anger, or constant stress can wire their brains to distrust others.

Toddlers need good food, affection, physical touch, play, and conversation to keep that growth on track. When midwives encourage parents to start talking to their babies and reading to them aloud starting at birth, that practice often continues into toddlerhood, strengthening both the brain and the bond between parent and child.

It was eye-opening for me to learn that in the Philippines many parents believe they don't need to begin feeding their children healthy foods until they start school. They reason that they need to feed their child's brain when formal learning begins, but they don't realize how early the process of brain development truly starts. Teaching about the first 1,000 days during pregnancy often comes as a revelation and transforms how families think about nutrition. Once parents understand that a child's brain is already 90% formed by the second birthday, they begin to see how crucial those early months are and how what happens long before school starts shapes a lifetime of learning and growth.

Now that we have seen how the first 1,000 days shape the developing brain, we can look at how this same period builds a foundation for lifelong health.

SAFEGUARDING THE CHILD'S HEALTH

The first 1,000 days set the foundation for health that lasts a lifetime. In recent years, scientists have deepened our understanding of how nutrition during the first 1,000 days shapes both immediate and long-term health. This early window influences the development of the immune system, affects future resistance to disease, and even impacts longevity.

Emerging research in epigenetics has revealed that the effects of poor nutrition can reach far beyond one lifetime. Nutritional deprivation leaves a biological imprint that can be passed from parent to child, influencing how genes are expressed in future generations. Studies of families who lived through famine show that their grandchildren still bear measurable effects of those early hardships. For this reason, our work to protect and nourish mothers and young children carries significance that extends across generations. The care we give today safeguards the health and potential of children and grandchildren yet to be born.

Let us now turn our attention to pregnancy and explore how health is built during this earliest stage of life.

HEALTH IN PREGNANCY

Everything that happens to a woman during pregnancy matters. What she eats, how she gains weight, her physical and emotional well-being, whether she is loved and cared for, the safety of her surroundings, and her daily habits all have a powerful influence on her child's future health. These influences reach far beyond what can be seen at birth.

During pregnancy, most of what is happening is invisible. A mother's nutrition and environment affect her baby's metabolism, immune system, and the development of vital organs. These same factors influence whether a baby grows to full term, is born prematurely, or is small for gestational age. Babies born at low birth weight often reveal signs of malnutrition that began long before birth, and these effects can last well into adulthood.

Research continues to uncover how adult diseases such as diabetes, hypertension, and cancer may have their origins during pregnancy. Prenatal nutrition, whether good or bad, appears to play a major role in determining a child's long-term susceptibility to these and other illnesses. While lifestyle and diet in adulthood still matter, of course, the roots of lifelong health may be traced back to what happens in the womb.

There is also fascinating evidence that babies may begin to develop food preferences even before they are born, shaping eating habits later in life. When nutrition is inadequate in the womb, a child may grow up with a greater risk of obesity and other metabolic problems, even if eating a normal diet after birth. These insights remind us that guiding mothers toward the importance of eating well during pregnancy is one of the most impactful ways we can care for the next generation.

HEALTH IN INFANCY

I cannot emphasize strongly enough the importance of teaching families about early and exclusive breastfeeding. Every baby should remain with the mother right after birth and begin to drink colostrum from her breast within the first hour postpartum. Establishing breastfeeding within this window, often called the Golden Hour, has been shown in research to lower infant mortality and improve health over a lifetime. The first hour is when a newborn possesses the most powerful instinct to find the nipple and suck. Colostrum, sometimes called liquid gold, is rich in antibodies, growth factors, and living immune cells that protect the newborn from infection and help seal the lining of the intestines. This first hour of extrauterine life has outsized and disproportionate importance in the overall course of a human life.

Breastfeeding lays the foundation for lifelong health and strong immunity, doing what no substitute or nonhuman milk can fully replicate. While other forms of milk can nourish a baby's body, it is the mother's milk that helps the baby build resistance to illness and grow strong.

Mother's milk is filled with antibodies, stem cells, and unique properties that respond directly to the environment, making it a natural form of personalized medicine. When a mother is exposed to an illness, her milk begins producing antibodies for that very sickness, often before she even feels symptoms, and her baby receives that protection. When a baby is sick, the mother's body gets signals through the baby's saliva to begin producing the perfect antibodies. This early immunity guards against common and deadly childhood diseases that still claim hundreds of thousands of young lives every year.

Breastfeeding also lowers a child's risk of developing a host of chronic conditions later in life. Even conditions like sudden infant death syndrome appear less common in breastfed babies. The evidence is clear that breastfeeding strengthens a newborn's health in countless ways, both as an infant and later as an adult.

Because of its power to protect health and save lives, many experts call breastfeeding one of the few true silver bullets in global health. The World Health Organization recommends exclusive breastfeeding for the first six months, beginning within the first sixty minutes after birth, and continuing into the second year if possible.

At six months, solid foods can be introduced while breastfeeding continues through the first year, and ideally, if possible, through the entire first 1,000 days, up to the child's second birthday. Many mothers face obstacles that make breastfeeding goals difficult to attain, from lack of support to the pressures of returning to work. But these goals remain worth striving for. The power of a mother's milk to nurture, protect, and sustain is one of the greatest gifts in the first 1,000 days of life. The best part is that if breastfeeding begins at birth and continues uninterrupted, the milk will continue to be produced, based on supply and demand, in just the right amount for years. And it is free!

MOTHER'S BENEFITS

The health benefits of breastfeeding extend to mothers as well. Research now shows that breastfeeding reduces a mother's risk of heart disease, diabetes, and certain cancers. When I began my midwifery studies in the late 1970s, I thought the benefits of breastfeeding were all for the baby. It was a gift I gladly gave to my own children. Over the years, I have come to understand that breastfeeding is not only lifesaving for babies but life-preserving for mothers as well. The process of breastfeeding is a truly symbiotic relationship, one that continues to bless me even now, 40 years later, by reducing my own risk for certain diseases as I age.

HEALTH IN EARLY CHILDHOOD

Building health continues into early childhood. We ideally want babies to receive breast milk for as long as mother and baby want to continue. During this time, along with nutritious food, a child needs to experience abundant love and family interaction. These early years are an opportune time to build lifelong health.

Early childhood is when habits take root that shape the rest of life. It is when a child learns what food means to them, what mealtimes feel like, and whether they associate nourishment with comfort and connection. It is also when they begin to form patterns of curiosity and learning, along with the sense of safety that comes from being loved and secure within their family.

AFFECTION AND INTERACTION

It is a universal truth that children need love. They need love they can feel and experience, with copious amounts of physical touch, affection, and attention. They need playtime with their caregivers and someone who will talk and read to them, even when they are too young to understand the words. The sound of a loving voice, the rhythm of speech, and the connection that comes through eye contact and gentle tone all help build positive pathways in a child's growing brain.

Even newborns benefit from hearing the familiar voices of those who love them. Holding, cuddling, and playing are not luxuries; they are essential for healthy emotional and cognitive development. These simple acts of affection and interaction lay the groundwork for future learning, helping children thrive in school and in life. Young babies are forming neural pathways at an astonishing rate, wiring their brains in response to every interaction.

Research in early childhood development shows that when a baby's needs are met with consistency and care, the brain builds pathways that reinforce security and trust. In the same way, when cries go unanswered and needs remain unmet, the brain may begin to encode patterns of stress and uncertainty, concluding that the world is not safe and that caregivers cannot be relied upon. These early synaptic connections, formed through repeated experiences, become the foundation for how a person will later perceive relationships, manage emotions, and respond to the world around them.

Reading aloud to a baby from birth is one of the simplest and most powerful ways we can teach parents to nurture brain development, and the effects can last a lifetime. Long before they can understand words, babies are listening to rhythm, tone, and the music of language, forming neural pathways that prepare them for speech and literacy. The warmth of a caregiver's voice during reading strengthens emotional bonds and reinforces the baby's sense of safety and belonging. If the book that is being read has pictures, the baby is also taking in colors and shapes, experiencing visual and auditory sensations. Reading books and singing lullabies can become moments of connection that shape both intellect and attachment, wiring the baby's brain for curiosity, learning, and trust. Ideally, every child should be read to daily until they reach school age and can learn to read on their own, and even beyond.

THE MIDWIFE'S ROLE

Approximately the first three hundred days of a child's life are within our purview as maternity providers. This is the time in the womb and about six weeks after birth. As midwives, we are in a powerful position to influence the remaining seven hundred days through our sharing of knowledge and encouragement. From the very first prenatal visit, we can start using the language of the First 1,000 Days to teach parents about the significance of this timeframe and help them understand that the choices they make now will shape their child's future health in body, mind, and spirit.

Even if our formal clinical role in a baby's life concludes shortly after birth, our voice of support can continue. Consistent wording and guidance, along with posters on the walls of our clinics and handouts reminding families about the first 1,000 days, can plant lasting seeds of awareness. Every conversation we have with an expectant mother or new parent can remind them that they hold a unique and precious opportunity to give their child the best possible start in life, and that this opportunity will never come again. In the human experience of the first 1,000 days, there are no do-overs.

OUR PHILIPPINE PROGRAM

Carmen, the bereaved mother I met on the road, was the catalyst for me to finally create a formal program to address a problem that had long weighed on my heart. With the help of our dedicated staff, we began to imagine what continued care could look like after a baby left midwifery care at six weeks after birth. When the Philippine government formally recognized the First 1,000 Days initiative in 2018, we knew the time had come to act.

What began as a pilot project soon grew into our robust First 1,000 Days program, which is now fully implemented across our birth centers in the Philippines. It is integrated with our preexisting midwifery services to provide holistic care throughout the entire first 1,000 days of a child's life.

We started by educating all our birth center staff on the concepts of the first 1,000 days, the same kind of information that you have been reading about in this chapter. Then we trained and employed women from the local communities around us to work beside our midwives and serve as home-visiting companions to families whose babies were born in our birth centers. We modeled this role after the community health workers used in many countries. We set their scope to cover the approximately 700 days after the birth and decided to call these auxiliary health workers Mercy Kasamas (*kasama* is the Tagalog word for "companion.") These Mercy Kasamas, or Kasamas for short, offer steady, personal support that is both practical and deeply relational. The Kasama meets the family during their prenatal visits to our birth centers, and helps with health messaging and childbirth classes. After the birth they begin a two-year journey of monthly home visits. Traveling by foot, motorcycle, or local public transportation, they visit homes in mountain villages, squatter settlements, and city neighborhoods to follow up on all the babies born in our Mercy In Action sponsored birth centers.

When they arrive for a First 1,000 Days visit, the Mercy Kasamas are warmly welcomed because they have already bonded with the family during prenatal care. They sit and talk with the parents, ask about the baby's feeding, play, and development, and encourage gentle, loving parenting. They support breastfeeding, guide healthy weaning, and teach the importance of nutrition using simple local foods. They weigh each baby monthly, chart the growth, and explain the concept of the "road to health," the normal weight-by-age range indicated by the curved lines on a child's growth chart. An upward climb between these lines means steady, healthy progress. A flat line is a warning sign, and we say a child "fell off the road to health" if their weight dips below the healthy range. In these cases, we employ interventions until the child is up on the road to health again, like supplementing the family's food supply, getting the child wormed, or treating underlying illness.

Mercy Kasamas do more than monitor physical growth; they also check developmental milestones at each month of age, and celebrate gains with the family. They look out for and address any concerns early. If a mother has stopped breastfeeding, they teach safe bottle feeding, and if a child gets sick, they are authorized to help with the cost of doctor's visits and medicines.

Mercy Kasamas support the family and nurture emotional connection and well-being by demonstrating baby massage, encouraging parents to read and talk to their infants, and reminding families that affection, play, and stimulation build strong, healthy brains. They teach about optimal child spacing and practical ways to protect children from harm or neglect. Each Kasama is trained to give special attention to babies who are small, premature, or struggling in any way, ensuring extra visits and follow-up care. All of this is connected back to our birth centers, where they report to the supervising midwife.

Thus, from the first prenatal visit through the child's second birthday, families receive continuous, integrated care from a team they know and trust. This holistic approach includes prenatal education, skilled birth care, postpartum support, breastfeeding guidance, parenting education, and physical and developmental monitoring.

Along the way, we mark milestones with special gifts for the child. Each baby born in our birth centers receives a special storybook at birth, to emphasize the importance of early reading. A pair of baby-size sandals is the gift on the first birthday, which is around the time most babies take their first steps. A birthday party with cake is how we celebrate the second birthday and "graduation" from the First 1,000 Days program. Years ago, I was told that the notion that a person isn't truly poor if they have at least one book and one pair of shoes is an expression of hope and dignity in Filipino culture. Hence the gifts of a book and a pair of shoes for each child.

Many of the babies in our program are born into extreme poverty. Without intervention, approximately one in every forty babies born in the Philippines will not live to see their second birthday. The First 1,000 Days program is that lifesaving intervention. It gives these babies a fair start, helping them stay on the road to health. It is a model of creative compassion and continuity of care that demonstrates how trusted caregivers, walking consistently beside families, can not only nurture physical health but also strengthen a child's chance to grow, thrive, and live out their full potential.

IT MATTERS FOR THIS ONE

Ceja was born in one of our birth centers as a low-birth-weight baby at just under five and a half pounds (2.5 kilos.) She entered the world small but full of promise, and luckily, her mother was committed to breastfeeding. Even so, when Ceja was one year old, she was hospitalized for an infection and came home weak and frail, having lost weight during her confinement. She fell off the road to health.

Ceja was receiving regular home visits from her Mercy Kasama ever since birth, so the family was given financial help to pay the doctors. It was her Mercy Kasama who noticed at her next visit that Ceja was still doing poorly, her weight still below the healthy range. Concerned, the Kasama put Ceja on her special care registry and began visiting more often, bringing bags of food at each visit to help the family improve her nutrition. With support from their Kasama, the parents focused on feeding Ceja extra meals each day, adding affordable, nutrient-rich local foods. The Kasama kept careful track of Ceja's growth and development through more frequent visits.

In time, Ceja began to regain her strength. Her energy returned, and her tiny cheeks grew round and rosy once more. With each visit, the family noted her steady progress on the growth chart and celebrated every small victory. Before long, Ceja was thriving again, back on the road to health and continuing to grow stronger each day.

The Talmudic teaching, "Whoever saves one life saves the world entire," comes alive in my heart every time we see a child recover from a dangerous illness, for each life we help preserve is a universe of possibilities, a story that might have been lost to the world. When we rescue even one child from the grip of poverty and malnutrition, we are safeguarding something priceless that extends far beyond what we can see.

Ceja's recovery reminds us why we do this work. The first 1,000 days offer an unrepeatable opportunity to build a foundation for lifelong health. In the past, we lost track of children like Ceja after they left our birth centers as healthy newborns. We now understand how important it is to keep walking beside the family, to be present when something happens that could push a child off the road to health. Even a short illness can cause dangerous weight loss, and being underweight at this stage puts a child at much greater risk of dying from a preventable disease. When we accompany families through those early days, we help shape a future where every child has the chance to grow, learn, and flourish. Babies have only one start in life. As midwives, we can take steps beyond our usual scope to make it a strong one.

CREATIVITY AND ENRICHMENT

My nineteen-year-old granddaughter Zoe came to the Philippines to spend half of her gap year with me after high school. A budding artist, she designed the artwork for a soft baby book that we printed on durable canvas. This small baby book project became a beautiful example of how creativity and enrichment can come together. Through Zoe's artistic gifts and her willingness to serve, every family who gives birth in our centers now receives a lasting reminder of love and thoughtfulness. Parents feel seen and cherished when someone does something special for their child, and these simple books inspire them to read to their babies from the very first days after birth. Though just a small project in the bigger scheme of things, it holds the elements that define our vision, purpose, strategy, and service; it is creative generosity expressed in a tangible way that nurtures both body and soul. Zoe made our First 1,000 Days program infinitely better with her creative gift.

As we close this section on the theme of creativity, I find myself feeling refreshed and renewed just by writing about the spirit of creativity that infuses everything we do in Mercy In Action. It nourishes my soul. I think of the words of Twyla Tharp in *The Creative Habit*, "A creative life has the nourishing power we normally associate with food, love and faith."

In Part III, we will turn our attention to the theme of generosity and examine our work in disaster relief, humanitarian aid, capacity building, and mission-driven education that improves health and healthcare for pregnant women and children even in the darkest places.

PAUSE FOR REFLECTION

WHAT BARRIERS KEEP MOTHERS FROM ACHIEVING THE BEST OUTCOMES FOR THEIR CHILDREN, AND HOW MIGHT YOU HELP REMOVE THOSE BARRIERS? HOW COULD USING THE PHRASE "FIRST 1,000 DAYS" HELP PARENTS GRASP THE LIFELONG IMPORTANCE OF THE CHOICES THEY MAKE IN PREGNANCY, INFANCY, AND EARLY CHILDHOOD? WHAT ARE SOME CREATIVE WAYS YOU COULD STAY INVOLVED IN PROMOTING GOOD NUTRITION AND STRONG EARLY CHILDHOOD DEVELOPMENT BEYOND YOUR TYPICAL SCOPE OF CARE?

PART III

A CULTURE OF SERVING WITH GENEROSITY

THE TRANSFORMATIVE EFFECTS OF EMPOWERMENT

A Tale of Newborn Survival: Rhonda's Story

This story is based on the experience of a newborn baby girl we cared for in the Philippines during my early years working in a sprawling urban slum in the capital city of Manila.

Rhonda was nearly dead when we found her, a three-week-old infant in the final phases of starvation. Weak, limp, and unable to move a muscle, she had spent the first weeks of her life in a dark and squalid hovel, one of thousands in the fifty-two-block maze of urban slum called Welfareville. Unable to suck since birth, her only nourishment had been the few drops of milk or water her parents occasionally dribbled down her flaccid throat.

They had other hungry children to feed, and no money to pay a doctor. I later learned that Rhonda was an unwanted child. As is all too common in places of extreme poverty, her mother had attempted to abort her during the pregnancy, using the primitive, crude methods known by despairing women in the slums. Rhonda was a survivor. She had survived the abortion attempt and three weeks of starvation and neglect. Now it was the morning of her twenty-third day, and Rhonda was barely hanging on.

That morning, my friend Kasey and I had come with a local midwife to this squatter area in Manila to talk to the barangay captain about setting up a health clinic. As we wound our way through the narrow, cramped maze of cardboard, tin, and scrap lumber houses, I heard a woman calling my name, asking me to please come and see her neighbor's sick baby.

She led us to a place that was hardly a house at all, just a gaping hole in the wall along the backside of the labyrinth of stacked dwellings. We had to step carefully to avoid the ribbon of raw sewage that crept through the narrow passageway, and the air hung thick and sour. Above us the shacks leaned together like a crooked tower of collapsing cards, sealing away the sun. Wires sagged between them and splintered boards jutted overhead, so that by the time we reached the doorway it felt less like walking down a street and more like crawling through a tunnel. A woman emerged from the dark hole and placed Rhonda in my arms.

I could see that the young infant was dying. Her physical presence in my arms was as light and insubstantial as a feather. Ribs protruded, wrapped in loose folds of ashen-gray skin. Tiny arms and legs dangled helplessly from her diminutive, wasted body. Her breathing was labored and shallow, and her sunken eyes were the only part of her body she could move. Rhonda looked up at me and made eye contact. In an instant, I knew that this ordinary day had just turned extraordinary.

We begged the mother to come with us right away to get her baby medical attention, but she refused. We asked permission to take Rhonda and do our best to save her life. The mother, seemingly resigned to her daughter dying, told us she did not want her and that we could do whatever we wanted. This was noted as highly unusual because even in cases of extreme lack, most mothers will do anything to help their babies survive.

I remember briefly thinking as we hurtled through the streets of Manila in a taxi that I could just drop this little baby off at one of the government hospitals in the city. No one would ever question that decision. No one would blame me. It was so tempting to just do that and give this awful responsibility to someone else. But I also knew that if I did, Rhonda would undoubtedly die. I had been working in hospitals for the poor in the Philippines and seen the conditions of overcrowding and understaffing. Parents are required to stay with their sick children for the entire hospital stay. If they accepted her for admission at all, without a family member to stay in the hospital with her, she wouldn't even get basic nursing care.

Back at the clinic, I inserted a narrow nasogastric tube down Rhonda's nose into her stomach and gave her tiny amounts of milk every fifteen minutes. We knew that since she was so dehydrated and starved, too much food at once could throw her into cardiac failure.

My son Ian was eight that year, and he and his two friends from Alaska, living with us that summer, were instantly enamored with little Rhonda, though she was smelly and had a skin infection all over her body, and an infected boil the size of a small egg on her little foot. I gathered Q-tips, soap, soft towels, and a basin of warm water, and showed Ian, Tabitha, and Brandon how to gently clean her sores. Tabitha asked if we should pray for her, and when I said, "Of course," she prayed like this: "Jesus, please don't let Rhonda die until she is a grandma."

I thought of the scripture about caring for "the least of these." There couldn't have been many who fit that description better than Rhonda did right then. As the kids prayed, I was visited with a deep sense of God's heart. He placed value on her—infinite, eternal value.

As gently as possible, I explained to the children that despite their ministrations and prayers, there was a good chance baby Rhonda wouldn't live through the night.

But Rhonda did live.

We fed her through the nose tube every few hours, day and night. It was touching to see how lovingly our children cared for the tiny, pitiful baby as they helped us treat her skin infection with ointment until it had cleared up. The other adults living in the clinic that summer took turns holding her close almost around the clock during the months she was recovering with us, knowing instinctively that Rhonda needed love as much as food. Most of all, we desperately wanted our human touch to give her the will to live.

Though we made every effort to support her parents to care for her, they seemed to have given her up for dead in the beginning of her life and would not take her back. Through a social worker, they released her for adoption. Any one of us caring for her in our clinic that year would have adopted her if complicated national laws hadn't prevented it.

For the first few weeks she was with us, Rhonda was too weak to cry, and after that she just never picked up the habit. She was always smiling, seeming happy simply to be alive. As she got older, we continued to offer her a form of kangaroo care, taking her everywhere with us in a baby sling strapped against one of our bodies. Back at home we exercised her arms and legs, sang to her, played with her, and read to her. When Rhonda was eight months old, she was finally able to drink from a bottle and eat mashed food, so she went to stay in a baby home run by missionary friends, where she was eventually adopted into a forever family.

My son Zak was thirteen years old that year; he loved her deeply, and he later wrote this about Rhonda for a school assignment:

> *When I was in the Philippines, several things made an impact on me, but none as great as a small little girl so weak and malnourished she couldn't even suck a bottle to survive. Her name is Rhonda. She enchanted me with her smile, moved me with her charming personality, and amazed me with her cheerful attitude. Every morning I would wake up early and go downstairs to see Rhonda grinning from ear to ear. Sometimes I would be in a terrible mood, and as I would walk by her playpen and accidentally look down to see her look up at me and laugh, I would forget everything and pick her up.*

Rhonda's story captured the hearts and imaginations of our supporters back in the United States. Hundreds of people followed her progress through our newsletters. Dermot Cole, a reporter for the Fairbanks Daily News-Miner, picked up the story and wrote articles about her. Rhonda became a symbol of hope for many, a mostly-dead, unwanted girl child from an impoverished Asian slum who survived against all odds. Little Rhonda, who started life with such profound disadvantage, found mercy and was given the chance to grow up and live a full life, maybe even someday becoming the grandma the children envisioned when they prayed.

9
CROSSING BORDERS

Women are not dying because of untreatable diseases. They are dying because societies have yet to make the decision that their lives are worth saving.

— DR. MAHMOUD FATHALLA

GENEROSITY HAS BEEN SAID TO BE ONE OF THE WAYS WE BECOME MORE fully alive as human beings. This is a concept well understood by people who choose to spend their lives giving of themselves to others. Thus, we begin the final section of this book by unveiling another secret to Mercy In Action's success in birth outcomes since the very beginning—a vision of excellent midwifery care offered in the spirit of genuine generosity to those who can least afford it.

Many midwives and others concerned with maternal and child health are sharing their expertise by taking on teaching and mentoring opportunities, going on mission trips, volunteering or working for nonprofit organizations, or even moving to a low-resource area to serve full-time. The best posture for this service is generosity that includes cultural awareness; freely sharing knowledge and building capacity among local midwives and healthcare workers will multiply the good work you are able to accomplish.

This chapter explores the awareness required of any midwife or birth professional to provide culturally competent care when entering a low- and middle-income country (LMIC), where neonatal and maternal mortality are high. By necessity, I am going to be generalizing, aware that while low-resource settings have different cultural attitudes and specific customs, there are still many similarities in the ways maternity care is experienced.

This chapter is organized around the ways things differ from what is familiar to readers in high-income settings in North America, Europe, New Zealand, and Australia. We will examine some of these differences across the prenatal, intrapartum, postpartum, and newborn periods of maternity care.

I believe that when we enter another culture, our role should be to strengthen local capacity and lead from behind, not to take over direct patient care. This form of humility and generosity honors native wisdom and builds sustainability. It is also the most culturally sensitive, culturally intelligent, and culturally humble way to serve.

THE INVITATION THAT BECAME A CALLING

I first received an invitation to serve beyond my own borders in the 1980s while I was running a birth center in Fairbanks, Alaska. This was previous to my being invited to offer help with maternity care in the Philippines. A Thai friend of a friend asked me to assist them in a maternal and child health project that they wanted to start in the country of Laos. Lamai ran an organization to help women escaping sex trafficking, and her husband had basic healthcare training as a medic. They hoped to expand their ministry into child survival and reach out into an area known as the Golden Triangle, where the borders of Thailand, Laos, and Myanmar (formerly Burma) meet.

During my time walking through markets in Thailand, I learned that the vendors use a charming expression when comparing two things that are similar yet distinct: "Same same but different." This expression fits here as the perfect phrase to reference as we begin this chapter on crossing cultures to find out how the provision of midwifery care may be "same same but different" from what we are accustomed to in our home countries.

PRENATAL CARE IN THE CONTEXT OF A LOW-RESOURCE, HIGH-MORTALITY COUNTRY

Same Same but Different

There are unique aspects to maternity care in a developing country, and while some prenatal care elements are universal, the midwife needs to be aware of how best practice can be different according to the setting.

Prenatal care, as well as the birth, should be free of barriers if we want to see change in the current poor outcomes of pregnancy globally. This means that a pregnant woman needs to be able to walk through your doors and be seen and evaluated without being required to pay first. During the initial prenatal exam, she needs to be assessed for any high-risk status and provided consultation or referral if needed. If she does not have the funds to pay for the care her situation requires, the midwife can help the woman navigate the maze of government or charity options for receiving maternity care in her community. This support is crucial to ensuring no one remains stranded without quality prenatal care as early as possible in pregnancy.

Food and Water

We realized very early in our work among those who struggle to meet basic needs that prenatal checkups alone were not changing outcomes. I have seen that nothing complicates a pregnancy as much as a mother not having enough to eat, and nothing improves pregnancy outcomes more than a well-nourished mother. Without a healthy mother there will not be a healthy baby; there is no getting around this simple equation. We include food as part of prenatal care whenever possible. For many years in Mexico and the Philippines, prenatal clinic day meant a large pot of nourishing soup simmering on the stove for the expectant mothers. When the setting does not allow us to cook hot food, we provide free prenatal vitamins to everyone, thanks to an ongoing grant from Vitamin Angels, and bags of food to malnourished mothers. We are aiming to strengthen the mother's health and, by extension, her baby's, while helping prevent many birth complications.

Midwives should screen all pregnant women in low-resource settings for malnutrition and wasting by measuring her mid-upper arm circumference (MUAC). MUAC is a simple and reliable way to assess a woman's nutritional status by measuring the circumference of her upper arm midway between the shoulder and elbow. It requires no special equipment other than a soft measuring tape. Studies have shown that both MUAC and a woman's pre-pregnancy weight are positively correlated with the baby's birth weight. These are essential screening tools that help identify women suffering from malnutrition so that interventions can be made early to prevent problems. We keep special registries for underweight patients who need regular food supplementation.

We must also remember the importance of safe drinking water. Potable water is essential for health during pregnancy, but it is often in short supply in many low-resource areas. As an alternative to the boiling of drinking water, over the years we have at times provided simple water filters, taught solar purification methods, and advocated for public use of clean water sources.

Laboratory

Certain laboratory tests are especially important for good pregnancy outcomes. In addition to the standard prenatal labs, women who live in areas where malaria, tuberculosis, or other local diseases are endemic should be tested for these conditions. In addition, anemia, urinary tract infections, and sexually transmitted infections must be treated as early as possible. It is also vitally important to screen for HIV and Hep B and Hep C. When these conditions are found and treated early, the chances for a healthy pregnancy and birth increase significantly.

Prevent Mother-to-Child Transmission

Screening for HIV/AIDS is not optional if we are to provide best practice prenatal care. Diagnosing and treating infections that can transfer to the baby during pregnancy, childbirth, or breastfeeding is one way to protect the baby from a deadly virus and increase the odds that the mother will survive and live to raise her child. Testing, treating, and supporting the mother must begin early in the pregnancy to be most effective.

In the 1990s our family helped raise an AIDS orphan whose mother died before he turned two years old. Juan had contracted HIV and hepatitis B from his mother in the womb at a time before there was prevention or treatment. It was a terrible, helpless feeling in those days before antiretrovirals came on the scene. We now have the medicine and the know-how to prevent mother-to-child transmission (PMTCT, also known as prevention of vertical transmission) of HIV/AIDS and hepatitis B and C, so that no mother need ever worry about passing these on to her baby again. We just need to be diligent to ensure that every woman gets tested and that those who test positive are treated.

Parasites

When someone asks me how midwifery differs in parts of the world that have limited resources, I often answer with one word: worms. That usually stops people in their tracks for a moment, as it is not the answer they expected. The medical term is helminths, and yes, they are a serious problem.

Anemia may be one of the first signs that we need to help a pregnant woman clear her body of parasites. The World Health Organization estimates that about forty-four million women are simultaneously pregnant and infected with hookworm. Hookworm is especially dangerous in pregnancy because it causes chronic blood loss, leading to prematurity and restricted growth of the baby in the womb.

Other parasitic infections also threaten maternal and newborn health. Schistosomiasis, which is caused by parasites that live in contaminated water, can damage internal organs and increase the risk of miscarriage and stillbirth. Roundworm and whipworm infections, both common in tropical regions, can worsen anemia and malnutrition in expectant mothers. These conditions, classified by the WHO as neglected tropical diseases (NTDs), remain widespread despite being preventable. Recognizing and treating them is an essential part of caring for mothers in the world's most vulnerable communities.

Warning Signs

You may be used to assuming that your client or patient will report any clinical problems they experience during pregnancy, even calling you on the phone if it seems serious. I have noticed that women in low-resource settings often do not report what they consider minor concerns until those concerns become major. Midwives are frequently not told about vaginal bleeding, severe headaches, or epigastric pain unless we ask directly during a prenatal visit. At times, these symptoms have been present for days, but the woman did not think they were important enough to mention to her provider. This may be because daily life is a constant effort to meet basic needs, which understandably demands most of their attention. They may also hesitate because they do not want to trouble the midwife. Delays in recognizing problems can be reduced through careful, routine questioning during prenatal care and by teaching the entire family a short list of key warning signs to report, any time of day or night.

Fundal Height

Textbooks commonly teach that a pregnant woman's fundal height should match the weeks of gestation, give or take two or three centimeters. But we began to question that standard in our setting, where many women are malnourished and smaller in stature. My niece Kate, a midwife trained in both the United States and New Zealand, was serving in the Philippines with Mercy In Action when she grew weary of sending laboring women to the hospital to deliver babies thought to be premature who turned out to be full-term at birth. In our birth centers, premature births are outside of a midwife's normal scope of practice, so when a woman's fundal height is measured low at the beginning of labor, it often appears she is not yet full-term and must deliver in a hospital. Without ultrasound or early prenatal records to confirm gestational age, these mothers were sometimes referred unnecessarily only to deliver healthy, full-term babies. In a culture where early prenatal care is not common and many women only access maternity care after labor has begun, fundal heights were the only way the midwives knew of to estimate gestational age.

Kate decided to lead a research project. She ended up studying 763 mother-baby pairs. Her findings confirmed that, in our unique low-income context in the Philippines, a fundal height of over 32 centimeters was correlated with a full-term baby 93% of the time. This simple but meaningful discovery demonstrated the need for localized standards. Similar studies could be repeated anywhere midwives serve women who are small-statured or chronically malnourished, to help establish a more accurate understanding of what is normal in that setting and to guide decisions about the safest place to give birth when labor begins.

Birth Spacing

In another Mercy In Action research project, this one conducted by my daughter-in-law Rose, we found that short birth spacing was a predictor of low birth weight in subsequent babies. Rose's research examined just one of the many problems inherent in short birth spacing for the newborn when the general health of the mother is compromised by poverty. This points to a need to focus prenatally on building health in mothers who are pregnant again before their previous child has reached two years old. It also highlights that we need to help mothers with birth spacing. We can do this best with protocols that encourage exclusive breastfeeding to six months postpartum, which in most women will delay ovulation. We can also make it a habit to discuss culturally appropriate family planning for safe child spacing, especially where birth control is not available, affordable, or acceptable.

Maternity Waiting Homes

In many countries, the mother can choose where to give birth; in others, home delivery is discouraged. For some women who are defined as "high-risk," staying near a medical facility for the end of pregnancy is the wisest choice. But many women with high-risk pregnancies have no relatives in town they can stay with and no money for a hotel. Maternity waiting homes are one solution. These are residential home-like structures located near a hospital or birth facility where women can await the birth of their babies. The presence of an affordable, culturally friendly maternity waiting home can make all the difference in safety and security as the due date draws near for an expectant family, as I described in chapter three.

Another use for these maternity waiting homes that we did not anticipate when we built them became to house women in late pregnancy who were severely malnourished and needed to receive food supplementation daily to get stronger before giving birth. By providing three solid meals a day, we worked to improve their health and reduce high-risk conditions before birth. This model can be used wherever the distance to a birth facility is too great and home birth is not an option.

Birth Preparedness and Complication Readiness Plan

Living and working in a place where many women and newborns don't survive birth forces the midwife to think differently about helping a family make prenatal birth plans. The way we address the three deadly delays is by recognizing the importance of a Birth Preparedness and Complication Readiness Plan. Every woman completes a readiness plan during her first prenatal care visit, and we review it at each subsequent visit to ensure she has a plan in place should the unexpected occur before, during, or after she gives birth. This was described in chapter five.

We must be deliberate about identifying and removing barriers to prenatal care. The midwives must be aware of the components that make up a strong foundation of care during pregnancy and maximize them to the best of our ability.

INTRAPARTUM CARE IN THE CONTEXT OF A LOW-RESOURCE, HIGH-MORTALITY COUNTRY

Same Same but Different

While many aspects of attending a labor and delivery are universal, the midwife needs to be aware that best practices can vary depending on the setting. The International Confederation of Midwives (ICM) has developed global standards, competencies, and guidelines to ensure that midwives worldwide have effective education and skills. When working in low-resource countries where maternal mortality and newborn deaths are high, the midwife should possess advanced skills such as administering IV antibiotics for sepsis, administering emergency treatment for eclampsia, and assisting birth with a ventouse as necessary for saving lives.

Although many births now take place in facilities, midwives with experience working outside of hospitals are especially suited to working in countries where home birth is the norm. Globally, fewer than half of all women have a skilled birth attendant present when they give birth. Many countries strongly encourage facility births, so Mercy In Action's midwife-led freestanding licensed birth centers serve as excellent alternatives to the hospital when home birth is not an option.

Barriers to quality midwifery care during labor and delivery must be removed worldwide. After facilitating access to skilled midwifery care, we must be aware of the components that make up a strong foundation of care during labor and delivery and maximize them. And we must realize that when labor begins, we may not have all the advantages that are standard practices in more developed regions of the world.

Risk Assessment in Labor

Depending on the setting, midwives do not always have the luxury of having prenatal records before labor begins. While lack of prenatal care is considered a risk factor by most practitioners, midwives working in a low-resource country must differentiate between risk factors and the actual risk posed to the woman or fetus right at the point you meet her in labor. This risk assessment once labor has begun is based on her vital signs, history, and rapid test lab results. In one of our inner-city clinics in Manila, more than 20% of births were to women we met for the first time in labor, because they had already been turned away in labor from one or more hospitals for lack of money. We learned to get very good at differentiating who had an actual risk that necessitated us doing everything in our power to get them into expert obstetric care, versus those who could safely deliver with us in our out-of-hospital birth center.

During the humanitarian crisis in the Philippines following Super Typhoon Haiyan/Yolanda, most of the women were unknown to us before they arrived at our disaster tents in labor. In these cases, it is essential for the midwife to do a rapid risk assessment and transfer out only those women who have a serious life-threatening condition that would necessitate a possibly Herculean effort to get the woman to an appropriate tertiary care hospital setting before the baby comes. In that disaster zone, the nearest functioning hospital was over ninety minutes away, and it was not operating at full capacity due to storm damage.

Rapid Lab Testing and Treatment

Lab tests you can do on-site at your facility during labor will help you determine your course of action to reduce risks if disease is present. These will include rapid tests for HIV and hepatitis B, as midwives can take special precautions in labor and at the birth to reduce the risk of mother-to-child transmission of these deadly diseases. Rapid tests are also available for syphilis, Zika, simple anemia, and more.

Grand Multiparity

Some midwives in high-resource countries work in communities where families routinely give birth to high numbers of children, but for most midwives, this is not the normal experience. It is important to be prepared for the unique risks that come with caring for grand multiparous women in labor (women who have previously borne five or more children), such as malpresentation, labor impediments caused by a pendulous abdomen or uterine exhaustion, and the increased risk of severe hemorrhage.

It is common in the Philippines for us to hear from a woman who has many children that her birth with us is the first time she has ever had a skilled birth attendant who offered her both emergency supplies and comfort measures. Almost without exception, a woman who says this to us will report after the birth that she loved the care and attention, not just the added feeling of safety and security.

Humble Surroundings

As a midwife who had my own planned home births in Alaska, I have always loved attending births in the home setting. However, home means something different for everyone. I was attending a homebirth conference in London in 1987 when I heard Sheila Kitzinger say not all homes are appropriate for safe birth, and I was taken aback. But when I began working in the slums of Southeast Asia shortly after that, I understood, because I saw firsthand that the housing conditions where many pregnant women lived and gave birth were shockingly lacking. Homes were often pieced together from scraps of tin and plywood, with gaps that let in rain and wind. Some had holes in the walls large enough for rats and pythons to wander in. Open drains carrying raw sewage ran through living spaces where mothers labored. Roofs leaked, floors were made of packed dirt, and livestock sometimes shared the room. I would like to say it is better now, but the poorest of the poor still live this way, and I still see it with my own eyes.

It is dangerous to romanticize these kinds of primitive birth settings. Neonatal tetanus still claims newborn lives, and when a woman gives birth on an unclean surface, she is also at risk of contracting tetanus or other deadly infections. Many times I have assisted a birth in homes with no indoor plumbing or running water, and often no proper bed for delivery. I once midwifed a breech birth on the narrow lower bunk of a sagging wooden bunk bed. And during a week of heavy monsoon rains, our midwives delivered a baby on the top bunk of a bunk bed in their living quarters because the clinic was flooding and they needed to keep mother and newborn safe and dry as the clinic filled with muddy water.

Infection Control

Over the years, I have heard comments such as, “Well, the surroundings are so dirty that things like carefully observing clean technique and sterile technique are not important.” In fact, the opposite is true. Where the risk of death from infection is high, we need to be extra careful to protect our mothers and babies, and in every way possible cut the risk of infection occurring during pregnancy, birth, or postpartum. A recent study showed that improving compliance with hand-hygiene standards and adopting evidence-based practices for infection prevention and management was responsible for a significant drop in infections. Written policy on how to detect sepsis early and deliver treatment using the FAST-M bundle (fluids, antibiotics, source control, transfer if required, and monitoring) has reduced deaths from infection by more than 30%.

Sacrum-Flexible Birth Position

Much has been written and taught on the benefits of upright birth, such as allowing gravity to help bring down the baby as well as avoiding the risk of hypotensive supine syndrome. Sacrum-flexible birth positions adds even more value to these benefits. A sacrum-flexible position is exactly what it sounds like: a position that allows the sacrum and coccyx (tailbone) to move freely backward, creating more space for the baby during birth. Unlike most of the bony pelvis, the sacrum is not completely fixed—it is designed to move. As the baby descends, the sacrum can tip backward and the coccyx can extend, increasing the diameter of the pelvic outlet. This added space can make a meaningful difference during the final stages of birth.

However, this natural movement is limited when a woman is in a lying down, semi-sitting or reclining position. In these positions, the sacrum is pressed into the bed, restricting its ability to move backward and reducing the available space for the baby. In contrast, positions such as sitting on a birth stool, squatting, kneeling, standing, hands-and-knees, or side-lying keep pressure off the sacrum and allow it to move as intended, making them optimal positions for a normal, physiologic delivery.

In settings where women may have a small pelvis due to a lifetime of under-nutrition, or are giving birth as teenagers before the pelvis is fully grown (the bony pelvis can continue to widen after general skeletal maturity, up to age twenty-five) we absolutely need to make sure the sacrum is able to open the pelvis to its largest possible opening to prevent obstructed labor. This slight adjustment to make an easier passage through the birth canal also lessens the stress on a baby who may not have been as well-nourished in the womb as we would like.

To help our birth-center midwives remember to encourage sacrum-flexible positioning during birth, I once used a simple demonstration. I pushed my way through our large glass clinic doors when they were only open a few inches. I managed to squeeze through, but not without obvious struggle—and a few bruises. As they watched, surprised and laughing, I said, "I can get through like this—but why wouldn't we just be generous and open the door a little wider so I can pass through comfortably?" That made the point. After that, they consistently remembered to support mothers into sacrum-flexible positions before the moment of birth.

Emergency Assisted Delivery

A midwife working in a high-risk setting must be prepared to assist with delivery when it becomes necessary to save a baby's life in cases of severe fetal distress or mildly obstructed labor, especially when hospital transport is not available or possible. It is wise for international midwives to learn how to use the ventouse. This tool is generally safer and easier to use than forceps in those rare but life-threatening situations when assistance is needed. When a midwife preparing to serve in a high-mortality region hesitates to learn ventouse skills, I remind them that this is never an alternative to a normal birth; it is an alternative to death. And it must only be used appropriately, with the sole purpose of preventing loss of life, never simply to hasten a delivery.

IV Antibiotics

In regions where group B strep (GBS) testing is not available, or in cases of unknown GBS status, if the mother has a fever of equal to or more than 38 C (100.4F) in labor, or has ruptured membranes more than 18 hours with birth not imminent, or her labor began earlier than 37 weeks, or she has a history of urinary tract infection (UTI) cultured as GBS infection earlier in the pregnancy, she needs to be given IV antibiotic treatment in labor as if she is GBS positive. A midwife's ability to recognize and treat GBS can mean the difference between life and death for babies.

Cultural Differences

A midwife working outside her own culture must take time to learn and respect the customs of the community she serves. At the same time, it is important to discern which traditions truly support the health and well-being of the family and which may cause harm. At times, the things we learn will be fun cultural traditions. At other times, the things we learn will feel harsh and unjust. For example, in some facilities, outdated rules and overcrowding prevent the woman from having a companion during labor. In some cultures, if a baby is born prematurely, it is said to be the fault of the husband, who must have had an affair. In other places, obstructed labor is thought to mean a woman must have been unfaithful, and she is shunned at the time she most needs loving assistance (and maybe professional help with an assisted delivery or cesarean). These are cruel beliefs with real-world consequences that lead to harm.

At other times, cultural values are just preferences. In some cultures, the male partner would not wish to attend the delivery, and it would be considered inappropriate for a male medical provider to care for a woman in labor. In many places, modesty during childbirth is a deeply held value that must be protected. Some cultures have specific foods a woman is expected to eat or not eat, and particular practices she should follow during labor.

Listening to the voices of local women through interviews and surveys helps us understand where change is needed and where practices continue to serve families well. Giving women a voice begins with asking thoughtful questions, truly listening to their answers, and creating space for their preferences to shape the care they receive when giving birth. It's important for us to be willing to learn with a spirit of curiosity rather than judgment.

POSTPARTUM CARE IN THE CONTEXT OF A LOW-RESOURCE, HIGH-MORTALITY COUNTRY

Same Same but Different

As is true with pregnancy and labor, so it is true of postpartum care: There are unique aspects to providing maternity care in a low-resource setting. While many recommended elements of caring for a woman in the period following birth are universal, the midwife needs to be aware of how best practices can be different according to the setting.

On one hand, postpartum care is the same everywhere, as we take into consideration the body that is healing after childbirth and the normal transition and growth of the newborn. It can also be very different. When working in developing countries where maternal mortality is high, the midwife should possess advanced skills and be humble about the high-risk population she may find herself among. Basic assumptions about how midwives deliver postpartum care may be challenged, and the scope of practice expected of the midwife may need to be redefined.

In most countries around the world, when measured against prenatal care and intrapartum care, postpartum is the most neglected period of maternity care, yet most maternal deaths happen in the postpartum period. Of all the postpartum deaths, approximately 45% happen within the first twenty-four hours after birth, and more than 65% within the first week. These sobering statistics remind us how critical the days and weeks after birth truly are and highlight the urgent need to strengthen postpartum care everywhere.

Cultural Expectations

The cultural expectations placed on a newly delivered mother are many and varied. Most cultures have specific foods a woman is expected to eat and certain things she is expected to do or not do during the postpartum period. Local customs often dictate where she lives, where she sleeps, and who cares for her and her baby. The length of the postpartum period also differs from place to place. In some cultures, special postpartum events take place within two weeks; in others, a woman may be expected to not leave her home at all for forty days.

A midwife caring for new mothers in a culture that is not her own must take time to learn about and respect the community's traditions, while also discerning which practices are beneficial, neutral, or harmful to the mother or baby. Hot soups after birth are good. Putting a coin under the pillow for good luck is harmless. A smoky fire kept under the bed of a mother and newborn in a small, closed room for weeks can cause harm. We learn to praise what is good, overlook what is harmless, and go slowly and gently with humility when addressing anything harmful. These conversations are best done in partnership with a bridge person who understands both healthy practices and the cultural meanings behind traditional practices. Most harmful practices are meant to protect the mother and baby, yet they can put their health at risk, so they must be addressed.

Preparing For After Birth

The midwifery model of care seeks to empower women and their families to thrive during the postpartum period, usually defined as the six weeks after birth. To do this well, educational materials are needed, and in many places, we have found that videos are often more effective than printed handouts. One reason is that even if someone cannot read, they can still understand a video. Another reason is that research shows many cultures place greater trust in information they have seen on television than in what a health provider tells them. To share vital postpartum information with new mothers and their families, create teaching videos or use those produced by nonprofit organizations such as Global Health Media. Their video "Caring for Yourself and Your Baby After Birth" is an excellent example.

Postpartum Warning Signs

While the danger signs after birth are the same all over the world, we must give special attention to those mothers who are in remote homes following childbirth with no phone or vehicle. They will need to be instructed carefully to alert someone who can drive them to a medical facility if they experience a complication. Just as we do with our prenatal Complications Readiness Plan, we give women a Warning Signs list to take home after birth, listing the serious postpartum complications.

Treating the Postpartum Big Four

All midwives working in low-resource countries must know how to prevent and manage the main causes of maternal death in the postpartum period. Globally, the leading causes of maternal death are hemorrhage, hypertensive disorders, infection, and obstructed labor. The first three of these can cause serious problems after birth, and the effects of the fourth continue into the postpartum period.

These complications are not always isolated events but are often connected, and it is common to experience more than one at a time postpartum. Bleeding at birth can increase the risk of infection later. High blood pressure after delivery can contribute to late postpartum hemorrhage by disrupting the clot at the placental site. Infection in the uterus can cause heavy bleeding, and obstructed labor can result in a fistula or the need for surgical delivery, both of which heighten the risk of infection and hemorrhage.

In many parts of the world, midwives are the ones responsible for administering antibiotics for sepsis and medically managing postpartum hypertension, especially in regions where the health system is overburdened. This reality highlights the need for midwives to have advanced clinical skills and confidence in their ability to provide lifesaving interventions rather than depending solely on referral to a physician or hospital.

Non-Pneumatic Anti-Shock Garment (NASG)

Death from shock following hemorrhage remains one of the leading causes of maternal mortality after birth. The simple device known as a Non-Pneumatic Anti-Shock Garment (NASG) is one of the things I would never want to be without when attending a birth. Made of neoprene, the same material used in a wetsuit, the NASG is a one-piece garment that wraps around the legs, pelvis, and abdomen and closes with Velcro. It has been included in the World Health Organization guidelines for proper treatment of postpartum hemorrhage since 2012 and is essential as an easy-to-use resuscitation tool for treating shock. The NASG works by safely redirecting a woman's own blood from her lower body back toward her vital organs, giving her core a kind of internal transfusion. Once the NASG is applied, we see remarkable changes. Her blood pressure rises, her pulse slows, her collapsed veins become visible for IV access, and her level of consciousness improves.

The NASG is a completely new design of the old military anti-shock trousers, much safer because it is non-pneumatic. The NASG was developed for use during home-to-hospital transport to stabilize a woman until she can receive a blood transfusion. However, in our experience at Mercy In Action birth centers in the Philippines, we have found that in more than half of the cases where the NASG is applied early in a postpartum hemorrhage, the mother stabilizes so no transfer is needed. We believe these positive outcomes occur because the NASG is used as part of a bundle of hemorrhage response, which includes oxytocin, fundal massage, and IVs, allowing us to protect the mother from progressing into severe shock.

The NASG has saved countless lives and remains one of the most valuable low-tech tools we have in maternity care today. It is relatively inexpensive, washable, and reusable up to one hundred times. Every provider of maternity care and every facility where babies are born would do well to have this lifesaving device.

Post-Birth Scoring Chart

As described in chapter six, we use the Post-Birth Scoring Chart we designed to screen our high volume of mixed-risk mothers in our birth centers in the Philippines to identify which risk factors are most likely to complicate their postpartum period. This chart helps us treat every mother after birth in an individualized way. It can help maternity care providers everywhere consciously evaluate what constitutes risks in the postpartum period based on what happened at birth so that they can provide extra care as appropriate.

Maternity Waiting Homes

Mercy In Action has also used the maternity waiting homes I described previously as safe places for postpartum families to stay for a few days after birth before hiking the long, steep trails back up to their mountain villages. Sometimes women have stayed a few days waiting for the river to go down after heavy rains, to avoid crossing when it is running more than waist-high and thus avoid a potential source of infection so soon after birth.

Occasionally, mothers who delivered in the hospital by cesarean also stay with us to recover before hiking home. One night, our caretaker heard an urgent pounding on his door; it was the husband of a young postpartum mother staying with us after she checked out of the hospital four days post-cesarean. He reported that his wife had suddenly started having severe difficulty breathing. Our ambulance was on site within minutes and whisked her back to the hospital, where she was diagnosed with a pulmonary embolism. If she had gone straight back to her village following the delivery, she might not have survived.

Postpartum Midwife

For many years we supported a midwife in Manila whose sole job was to visit all the mothers who had given birth in a large slum area, to assist them with postpartum recovery, breastfeeding support, and medical care as needed. The women welcomed this visiting midwife who came around after they were discharged from the local hospitals, as it was the only postpartum follow-up care they received. The families expressed how much they appreciated the midwife model of postpartum care and the relationship that came with it. We helped new mothers and babies thrive by not limiting our postpartum care to only those who gave birth in our facilities.

NEWBORN CARE IN THE CONTEXT OF A LOW-RESOURCE, HIGH-MORTALITY COUNTRY

Same Same but Different

There are unique aspects to caring for babies in low-resource settings, and while many parts of the six weeks of follow-up after birth are universal, the midwife must understand how best practices differ depending on the context.

In developing countries where neonatal mortality (up to 28 days old) is high during the early weeks of life, the midwife must have advanced skills and a deep humility about the high-risk populations they serve. Some Western cultural attitudes may be challenged; we will have to think differently.

Small Babies

It is sad but true that there is often not enough food for pregnant women to eat during pregnancy in low-resource areas. Thus, babies are more likely to be born small for gestational age or to experience intrauterine growth restriction. At times, we care for babies who were born early if there is not a hospital with a neonatal intensive care unit (NICU) available. A great resource for learning how to care for these babies is a course called Essential Care for Small Babies, part of the Helping Babies Survive modules endorsed by the WHO.

Sepsis

Treatment of newborn sepsis may be part of your midwifery job description. You may have always referred a baby to a pediatrician if you suspected infection, but now you need to learn to administer antibiotic injections or IV treatments yourself to save a newborn's life. These and other skills can be learned by taking extra training, such as that offered in the Helping Babies Survive series mentioned above.

Disease Risk

Babies born in countries where preventable diseases are still prevalent are too often maimed and killed by illnesses that can be prevented with immunizations. Some vaccinations are given at birth and others during the first weeks and months after birth, and immunizing babies is often part of the midwife's job description. For those who have never seen diseases such as polio, tetanus, or measles firsthand, it is important to understand the burden of disease and offer parents fully informed consent and sound guidance for their children, who may be at great risk.

The toll of preventable childhood disease affected my own family in a deeply personal way. My late husband contracted polio as a little boy in Montana, one year before the polio vaccine became available in the United States. One night he went to bed a healthy five-year-old child and woke up the next morning with paralyzed legs and excruciating pain. My mother-in-law told me that in the 1950s, every parent feared the summertime when polio cases would break out, causing widespread paralysis and thousands of deaths, until the introduction of a vaccine in 1955 drastically reduced cases. Scott made a recovery, but the polio virus's painful effects returned later in his life as post-polio syndrome, reminding our family that behind every vaccine-preventable disease, there is real suffering that may last a lifetime. We don't see these diseases much in high-resource countries anymore, but they are still very much a threat in areas where immunization rates are low.

Preventing Mother-to-Child Transmission

In places where midwives are the primary care providers, they may be called upon to provide immediate treatment to newborns who are born to mothers with hepatitis B or HIV. In this case, immunization is not a routine precaution but a lifesaving act to prevent the transmission of a deadly disease from mother to child. Hepatitis B is endemic to the Philippines where I live, as it is in other countries as well. When a mother tests positive for Hep B infection during our prenatal care, or during rapid testing at the time of her arrival in labor, the preventative treatment is for the baby to receive the first vaccine against Hep B right there in the delivery room. Babies born to carrier mothers face a higher risk of infection during birth, but they can be protected by receiving both the vaccine and immunoglobulin for Hep B (HBIG) soon after delivery. When the full series of vaccines is completed, the baby's risk of infection drops by about 95%. As a bonus, while Hep B is incurable in the mother, we can educate her on wellness choices that can allow her to stay healthy longer so she can raise her child.

With an HIV-infected mother, we need to start further back by starting antiretroviral treatment during pregnancy, as well as giving a dose during labor, to protect the baby from contracting HIV from the mother. Then the baby should continue to receive doses after birth, under the supervision of the midwife and a team of medical providers dedicated to keeping her alive and the baby free from mother-to-child transmission.

Pregnant mothers being diagnosed with Hep B, Hep C, or HIV/AIDS is not just an abstract concept to me. I have seen firsthand the suffering these viruses can cause. I lost two friends to liver damage from hepatitis B. One of them was in his early thirties, and had been infected at birth through mother-to-child transmission. And I have experienced the heartbreak of caring for young mothers with AIDS who did not live to raise their babies.

A missionary midwife once told me, "I am against all immunizations." I remember thinking that due to the dangers of hepatitis B passing to an innocent baby, we do not have the luxury of making such sweeping statements. Even if a provider feels hesitancy about all the prophylactic vaccinations available, we need to be clear on which ones are directly preventing a current disease from spreading to a newborn, as well as which diseases are widespread in the area you are serving. Midwives who understand the importance of testing and early treatment hold in their hands the power to protect a new generation from diseases that take far too many lives too soon.

Early and Exclusive Colostrum

The timing of initiating breastfeeding right after birth is critical not only for health but also for survival. Research has shown that babies who receive colostrum within the first hour after birth have the lowest risk of death. Every hour that passes without latching and drinking colostrum increases that risk. It is a direct relationship: The more time passes without nursing, the more the risk of neonatal death rises. Babies who are given any non-human milk in the first few days after birth are four times more likely to die than babies exclusively breastfed. Large studies involving more than thirty thousand babies in Nepal and Ghana confirmed these findings. We can extrapolate that health in general is going to be the very best possible if breastfeeding is early and exclusive in all newborn human babies.

My daughter-in-law Manga asked an important question in her master's research study, first posed in her title, "Is the Birth Attendant a Risk Factor for Delayed Initiation of Breastfeeding and Non-exclusive Colostrum?" The answer she found was a resounding yes. Studying births attended by doctors, midwives, and traditional healers in different settings such as hospitals, birth centers, and homes, she found that it is the birth provider's attitudes, not about breastfeeding in general, but about the importance of early colostrum, that determine whether a baby actually starts nursing soon after birth. The person responsible for the delivery must intentionally keep distractions and disruptions surrounding the moments after birth to an absolute minimum so the baby can nurse undisturbed and receive the powerful effect of colostrum in the first hour.

The Golden Hour

The hour immediately following birth is known as the Golden Hour because of the unique physiological readiness of newly born babies to latch on and begin nursing, and because the impact of receiving colostrum during this time sets the course for better health throughout the baby's life. Newborns are born with a strong instinct to find the nipple and suck, but it diminishes toward the end of the first hour after birth, and after that it must be learned. As midwives and birth professionals, we must ensure nothing hinders that early breastfeeding. Within that first hour when colostrum flows from mother to child, a foundation for lifelong health is being built, and bonding between the parents and baby is happening, both of which are necessary for a baby to thrive in this life. Therefore, if the baby is breathing at birth, nothing else is a higher priority than letting that newborn nurse for the first time within the sixty minutes right after birth.

The First 1,000 Days

We have learned in chapter eight that, for the best outcomes, care and monitoring of the newborn should ideally extend beyond the traditional six weeks after birth to encompass the entire first 1,000 days of life. As long as pneumonia, diarrhea, malaria, measles, and malnutrition remain among the top causes of death for young children in low-resource communities, we will closely monitor our babies until they turn two years old.

Honor the MotherBaby-Family Triad

Remember that what is good for the mother is good for the baby and good for the family, and never more so than when families are under duress due to poverty. We must do everything possible to encourage strong bonding at birth and to keep them together afterward.

Even though in writing this chapter I needed to separate postpartum and newborn care into two sections, in practice the mother and baby are always cared for together and should be viewed as one unit. The best resource for training midwifery staff on this essential but often underappreciated concept is the International Childbirth Initiative (ICI) 12 Steps to Safe and Respectful MotherBaby-Family Maternity Care. The visionary authors of the 12 Steps coined the term MotherBaby, written with a capital M and B and no space between them, then added a hyphen to connect to the word *family* to show the sacred unity of this human dynamic.

This understanding of seeing maternal and newborn care as interconnected and relational is at the heart of why our outcomes are so good. When mother, baby, and family are supported and valued as one, the mother's recovery is quicker, the baby's chances for survival improve, and the family bond grows stronger. We have seen time and again that when we protect this unity, even in the most difficult circumstances, the results are life-giving.

Parenting Advice

In addition to the usual advice midwives give new parents, there are a few other important considerations in this context. Parents should be encouraged to keep the baby and the mother under a treated mosquito net in regions where malaria is common. If cooking or heating is done over an unventilated fire, remind families to protect the newborn from inhaling too much smoke. For mothers taking antiretroviral medicine for their positive HIV status, stress the importance of giving their newborns their daily treatment as well.

Teach parents to recognize danger signs in a newborn, such as rapid breathing, lethargy, or lack of interest in nursing, and to seek help immediately from a qualified health professional rather than turning to harmful traditional practices. More than once I have seen newborns with holes burned into their tiny ankles by well-meaning traditional practitioners trying to "let the bad out." While we strive to understand why people do what they do, we still have to correct harmful practices when we see them, and teaching parents the right way to care for a baby is paramount.

In low-resource areas, breastfeeding is not simply one feeding option among many; it is a vital lifeline for a newborn's survival. We must work diligently with any mother who struggles to breastfeed, especially those living in situations of poverty where formula feeding does not meet the criteria known by the acronym AFASS—acceptable, feasible, affordable, sustainable, and safe. The guidance you offer in this situation can truly make the difference between life and death for a baby.

RESPECT AND AUTONOMY

Disrespectful treatment during labor is now clearly defined, categorized into behavioral types, and closely monitored by human rights organizations. At Mercy In Action birth centers, we place a high value on respect and patient autonomy, modeling these principles in every interaction with the families we serve. We not only teach respectful care but also hold ourselves accountable by voluntarily using the International Childbirth Initiative women's questionnaire, which mothers complete after birth to share whether they felt treated with dignity and respect. Respectful maternity care has rightfully become an essential part of culturally competent practice, and each of us is called to understand what respect looks like within the specific culture where we serve.

RESPECT NATIONAL HEALTHCARE LAWS

National healthcare laws must always be respected. One of my Filipina midwife friends once recalled being reminded by a government official, "Ignorance of the law is no excuse for breaking the law."

That truth applies even more so to foreign volunteers who travel abroad to practice midwifery. Most countries have a formal process for obtaining prior approval before offering any kind of medical service, ensuring that any volunteering that involves providing healthcare is carried out both legally and ethically.

In the Philippines, this process includes obtaining a temporary permit from the Professional Regulation Commission (PRC) if a visiting healthcare provider plans to perform any medical services beyond observing or assisting a locally licensed doctor or midwife. In the event of a global pandemic or major natural disaster, standard local licensure requirements may be temporarily waived; however, a valid license from your home country will still be required.

LEADING FROM BEHIND

The concept of leading from behind is a powerful strategy that does not break any laws anywhere, and it is generous because it helps local providers gain the confidence they need to lead. Nelson Mandela once said that a good leader is "like a shepherd. He stays behind the flock, letting the most nimble go out ahead," and then gently guides the others to follow.

Leading from behind, rather than seeking the glory of delivering babies yourself, is the generous choice. It also protects a foreign midwife from potential legal charges of practicing midwifery or medicine without a license. At Mercy In Action's sponsored birth centers, our strategy is to not have foreign workers provide direct patient care and instead we focus on training national midwives and community health workers. We choose to lead from behind as we teach, empower, and build capacity among local midwives wherever we work.

This approach of leading from behind is both humble and forward-looking. It represents generosity and cultural intelligence, and it is what we believe the future of medical volunteering in low-resource settings must become—a sustainable model rooted in respect and empowerment.

The one exception to this principle is during immediate disaster response, in which case the government of the country affected may open the borders to foreign aid workers to serve until their own healthcare workforce can get back on their feet. Even when we are assisting after disasters, however, we hire local midwives as soon as we can identify them. After the crush of the first wave of disaster response is over, we work to help the local midwives rebuild and get their own birth centers open again as soon as possible.

GENEROSITY OF SPIRIT

Midwives are known for going above and beyond the call of duty to ensure the safety of mothers and babies in their care. Maternity care in the context of poverty will make even more demands on your time, your resources, and your wallet. It may require more of your heart and soul than you thought possible to give away. However, on this point, I agree with what Dr. David Livingstone said when he was speaking at Cambridge University toward the end of his life in 1857. He was asked to address the many great sacrifices he made throughout his life as a medical missionary and antislavery advocate. "Away with the word 'sacrifice,'" he said. "Say rather it is a privilege."

There are many cultural ways people approach healthcare during the childbearing journey. We should always seek to understand how our various cultural lenses shape our feelings, thoughts, and actions. In all we do, we should seek to be guided by a generous desire to serve the mother, the baby, and the family in ways that honor their dignity and best interests. If we allow ourselves to love to the full extent of the grace given to us in difficult situations, our work in international maternity care will make a lasting difference in both mortality and morbidity outcomes and will bring rewards beyond measure.

Birth doesn't pause for crisis, and midwives are sometimes called upon to bear witness to great suffering, chaos, and danger in the call of duty. Babies will continue to be born even during the terrors of natural disasters, wars, and crushing poverty. In the next chapter, we will examine midwives' responses in the wake of such disastrous situations.

PAUSE FOR REFLECTION

When you serve in a culture that is not your own, how can you enter as a learner first, before offering your own experience? What specific ways can you strengthen local capacity by teaching, mentoring, and sharing skills that empower national midwives to lead sustainable change? How will you discern whether your presence is helping to build local ownership of maternity care, or unintentionally taking the place of those who should be leading the efforts?

10
BUILDING CAPACITY AMID DISASTER AND POVERTY

No one has ever become poor by giving.

— ANNE FRANK

AFTER BARELY SURVIVING THE PHILIPPINES' SUPER TYPHOON ON November 8, 2013, and being terrified for hours as she and her young family struggled to keep their heads above water and not be crushed to death, Nerissa Cumpio looked out at dawn the next day on a world she did not recognize. She later told me that her first thought was, "Is this still planet Earth?" Every building, every familiar landmark, was destroyed and lying in rubble. Even the hills were deforested, all the trees lying down or snapped off at mid-trunk in grotesque, twisted shapes. Leyte Island was unrecognizable.

Responding to warnings the night before, they had shuttered their birth center after the last patient left and headed away from the coast to a relative's home as the typhoon approached, but the storm surge, along with winds blowing almost 200 miles per hour, reached farther inland than anyone had predicted and trapped them in a nightmare. It destroyed everything in its path, and they were lucky to survive.

As Nerissa and her husband Alex climbed over the rubble to return to their home, she witnessed people carrying dead bodies, and she saw yet more bodies lying in the streets, on the beach, askew in the broken branches of a tree. It was an unfamiliar world of death and destruction.

Nerissa held their four-year-old daughter, who was traumatized and shivering with lips turned dark blue from having been submerged in the flood waters for so long. Alex walked ahead of her, holding the hand of their older daughter. She wondered if they would survive the aftermath of this destruction. It was slowly dawning on Nerissa and Alex that all the clean water sources were contaminated with seawater, and there was no food to be had. But the worst was yet to come.

As they got closer to home on the coast, to their horror, they began to recognize some of the dead bodies. They came upon neighbors and friends carrying the remains of people they had known and loved. By the time they reached the broken cement that was all that remained of their home and birth center, they could barely go on, exhausted, heartbroken, and close to despair. As family members still alive began to find one another and tearfully reunite, they realized no one had any means to help anyone else anymore.

A few days later, after having received a tarp for temporary shelter and standing in lines for hours to receive a meager daily rice handout from the first responders who had started arriving, Nerissa went to check on her patients. Of course she did; she was the community's midwife, and it would have never crossed her mind not to feel responsible for the patients in her care.

One patient she found, Belinda, related through sobs that the baby Nerissa had helped her deliver a short time before was gone, torn from her arms by the wind and waves, washed out to sea. They cried together. There were other stories like that, other mothers and fathers to comfort, and pregnant women to visit, even though Nerissa no longer had any equipment to check blood pressure or measure a fundal height or listen to the beat of a fetus's heart; all her midwifery equipment washed out to sea as well.

One day Belinda sought Nerissa out to tell her about a dream she had the night before. "In the dream, I was pregnant, and your birth center was rebuilt, and you helped me deliver my baby there." Nerissa smiled sadly at her friend, but to herself she thought bitterly, "Look around. Everything is destroyed...that dream is not going to happen."

WHAT WE CHOOSE TO GIVE AWAY

This chapter is divided into two main parts. The first part is about generous investment in building clinical capacity in areas of extreme disaster or ongoing poverty. The second part is about generous investment in sharing knowledge with other birth workers and outreach to communities through learning opportunities they would not otherwise have. Examples will showcase creative ideas for generous capacity building using a variety of teams and settings. All this connected to our larger vision of improving birth outcomes for everyone, everywhere, being mindful of how hard it can be to survive birth when the world around you is broken.

DISASTER ON DISASTER

At the time Super Typhoon Haiyan (known locally as Yolanda) hit Leyte Island, we were still recovering from massive flooding in northern Luzon Island, where I live. The cement foundation of our birth center had been seriously damaged by a flood in September, which cost thousands of dollars to repair. My own home had flooded in another storm ten days later when 90% of our town went underwater. That night we had barely gotten Scott's ninety-year-old mother up the stairs into the storage space before the waters overtook the first floor of our little house. Trying to save important papers, books, and electronics, I found myself swimming through dirty river water over my head inside our home. Little did I know until a week later that I had contracted leptospirosis in the flood waters, one of hundreds of people caught up in the epidemic that swept through our community on the heels of the flooding. I was still recovering from this painful zoonotic disease when we heard the news of the destruction and devastation in the islands to our south. Though typhoon season had been particularly rough on us that year, it quickly became apparent from the news that our neighbors down south were hurt much much worse.

Reports were of complete infrastructure collapse. There was nowhere to take the injured because the hospitals and clinics were destroyed. Early scenes we saw in the news were of desperate mothers giving birth in rubble inside broken buildings and along highways. I remember seeing a picture in the newspaper of two newborn premature babies lined up on the altar of a damaged church, wrapped in plastic bags to keep warm, and thinking someone needs to tell them to use kangaroo care. Headlines blared "High Birth Rate Strains Philippines Recovery Efforts," and NBC ran a piece called "Born into disaster: 12,000 babies on the way in Philippines' typhoon-stricken region." I was getting firsthand accounts from a former Marine friend already down there, who said it was mass chaos. Rose called me and summed it all up in one statement when she said, "Vic, we have to respond." I knew it was true.

There is never a good time for a disaster, so although our organization's finances and my health were not in the best of shape, we packed up and went to deliver babies in tents for the next few months. Our decades-long commitment to altruism, our understanding of disaster response best practices, and our proximity compelled us to quickly mount a relief effort on a scale far larger than anything we had done before.

ALTRUISM

Defined as the kind of love that gives freely without counting the cost, altruism means acting for the good of others without expecting anything in return. This kind of love is possible if our actions are tied to our purpose and motivated by something greater than ourselves.

This chapter is about generosity that transcends walls and crosses borders, both metaphorically and literally. In the worst possible conditions amid humanitarian disasters, midwives will always be desperately needed on the scene, as every population has a percentage of people pregnant at any given time. Babies are still due to be born, and the trauma of disaster often sets off labor in women who are close to their due dates, or causes premature labor due to the stress. But whether the disaster is natural and strikes without warning, or caused by war, refugee crises, or extreme poverty, midwives will at times be called upon to set everything else aside and respond, because it is in our hearts and within our skill sets to do so.

The kind of altruistic responses I describe in this chapter are based on capacity building rather than a one-off handout. Altruism as we practice it seeks to respond to the urgent needs and also rebuild stronger for the future. Disasters can happen anywhere. As midwives and those who support midwives, we must respond to what befalls us, but we can also choose to go into someone else's disaster to help, because it will improve the birth outcomes in places hardest hit.

THE DREAM COMES TRUE

Ten months after this deadly storm hit the Philippines, Nerissa Cumpio and I stood shoulder to shoulder, gripping a pair of large scissors as we cut the ribbon to open her rebuilt birth center. With grants and donations from good souls all over the world, Mercy In Action rebuilt the Cumpio Birth Clinic from the ground up, and furnished and stocked it with supplies. Smashed beyond all recognition in the typhoon, it rose like a phoenix from the ashes, and less than a year after being destroyed, the doors opened with a new license to operate, and just like that, babies were being born there again.

Belinda gave birth in this bright new birth center only three weeks after the grand opening, attended by her friend and midwife Nerissa. It felt like a miracle to them both, in a space only dreamed about in the terrible weeks and months following the disaster. Belinda's literal dream proved prophetic; life unfolded just as she had seen it, and she had a new baby boy in her arms.

A COUNTRY OF DISASTERS

Out of necessity, Mercy In Action had incorporated disaster planning into our Philippine maternity care from the very beginning. My first year in the Philippines was 1991, and I was asked to offer healthcare after the eruption of Mount Pinatubo displaced large numbers of indigenous people known as the Aeta. Over the years, we responded to many disasters: volcanoes, earthquakes, typhoons, floods, and fires. While working to help our patients in a holistic way, we learned how best to help a community recover from disasters big and small. Eventually we began teaching our own disaster preparedness course for midwives and other health workers, responding as crises happened around us. All this was long before Haiyan/Yolanda forced us into a disaster response on a much larger scale.

LOGISTICS

To respond to the Haiyan/Yolanda disaster, our entire team went into action. Our logistics team, led by my husband, Scott, loaded our ambulance with birth supplies from our northern birth center on Luzon Island, and added tents, beds, water filters, canned tuna and Spam, noodles, and rice. All this was driven and then ferried to ground zero of the disaster zone on Leyte Island, a difficult two-day journey away. We were fortunate to have our own ambulance and driver, as only emergency response vehicles were being allowed to cross onto Leyte Island at that time.

I led the midwife team. A runway had been cleared of rubble at the airport in the capital, right before I flew in with two of our local midwives and two other helpers. Jack, the former Marine friend I mentioned earlier, met us down there. Climbing onto the roof rack of our ambulance at the airport because there was no room inside, perched on boxes of supplies, we drove out of the capital to reach the hardest-hit area. As the sun set on our small team that first night, we set up a living quarters tent and a private medical tent. Our team slept on the ground and saved the beds for the patients.

Three days later, Rose flew in from the USA with a large sheepherder tent she purchased in Idaho, to be used as our delivery room for the next several months. Airlines all along her route had given her free oversized luggage allowance in solidarity with the survivors of a storm that was still being reported nightly in the world news.

SCOPE AND PRIORITIES

Looking back now on our immediate disaster response to Haiyan/Yolanda, the scope of maternity care and medical services we were able to provide still humbles me. In that short season, we provided the midwifery model of care in a disaster tent for 116 deliveries. We gave each woman a private, safe, and respectful birth despite the tight space and privation all around us. Even though every pregnant woman we cared for was living in terrible conditions without enough to eat and no electricity or running water, there were only two perinatal losses among our hundreds of patients during that time. The first loss was to a woman who arrived to our tent in labor with her baby already dead inside her, and later another baby died at eight days after birth from an unknown cause.

Feeding people who were starving was a priority, and we achieved this in our area of responsibility through partnerships with other agencies and NGOs. We enrolled 367 pregnant women in ongoing prenatal nutritional support, and 648 breastfeeding women in our postpartum feeding program, providing the calories they needed to continue growing and nourishing their babies.

During the first two months, we provided wound care to another 1,532 non-pregnant people, cleaning and suturing lacerations, especially on hands and feet. We administered tetanus toxoid immunizations around the clock, as people were injured constantly while continuing to dig in the rubble to find bodies of loved ones throughout this entire time. We used our ambulance to transport people experiencing various emergencies, and on occasion, we were pressed into service to treat asthma and other ailments worsened by the inhospitable environment.

Although we were working to ensure babies were born safely under extreme conditions, we held firmly to the steps of Baby-Friendly and Mother-Friendly care, believing that best practices in maternity services should be the standard for disaster care, just as in any other setting. Every service we provided was given freely, including essential medicines. We also shared our supplies with other healthcare providers in the disaster zone, and other groups shared theirs with us.

Knowing the risk of post-traumatic stress disorder to our patients and our first responders, we strategically invited spiritual counselors to join us. Virmi, a dear Filipina friend from Manila trained in trauma counseling, joined us and was invaluable in the early days of our response. We held daily trauma-healing seminars attended by hundreds of adults and children, where people were given space to grieve and process in a structured way. After Christmas, Kristen's mom, Jamie, an ordained chaplain, flew over with Matt to serve the ongoing spiritual needs in our tents. All in all, thousands of survivors were prayed for by our team as we bore witness to their trauma, grief, and loss.

PARTNERS

Mercy In Action partnered with Doctors Without Borders for transport to their tent hospital, as needed, for the rare cesarean (2% of our births), and USAID provided high-protein food supplements for our pregnant and nursing mothers. From UNICEF, we received a large tent designated for breastfeeding support, which we used to provide long-term care for mothers of premature babies and twins who needed 24-7 kangaroo care. We forged other partnerships with groups like Samaritan's Purse, who enrolled all the malnourished children of our maternity patients in their feeding program, bringing the food to our tents for us to distribute.

It was a time of incredible global cooperation with a single-minded focus of helping a people who were badly hurt and had no means to help themselves. The World Health Organization set up headquarters in the capital to coordinate our efforts, which was invaluable for establishing partnerships. At the broken airport, military planes from dozens of countries crowded the runway, their flags painted along their sides, each one marking a distant nation that had come to help in the wake of the catastrophe. I was told when we needed supplies that I could ask anyone at the airport in military uniform. So one day I walked out onto the tarmac and approached a Philippine Air Force officer, who allowed me to climb into the transport plane he was loading and hitch a ride to another island untouched by the disaster. I was the only civilian on board, standing up, squeezed in the cargo bay on the short flight. After I bought a generator, a small fridge, and a large quantity of medications, I caught a ride back on another military transport plane. This kind of experience was common during that time of unusual cooperation between the governments of the world and the hundreds of NGO personnel from dozens of global organizations responding to the disaster.

Our financial partners were heroic throughout Mercy In Action's ongoing response to this crisis. Individual donors and a few churches funded everything we needed to function at a high level of excellence in our disaster tents, and the supplies never ran out. We had enough to use and share with other responders. Since no other organization delivering babies in the disaster zone had the NASG for postpartum hemorrhage, Scott ordered a large shipment from China and we trained the staff of Doctors Without Borders, the Red Cross, and many local midwives on how to use them. After the training, we donated an NASG to every temporary facility we knew of that was delivering babies in the disaster area, and made sure each local midwife had one.

I would be remiss not to mention how much my own family amazed me by stepping up to help during this time of extreme distress while I was physically in the disaster zone. I already mentioned that Scott ran the logistics from our home on the island of Luzon. My sister and my parents coordinated shipments of supplies and made sure we never ran out of vitamins to distribute. Sean, a doctor by this time, left his work in California to come and serve in our tents alongside our team. Zak and his wife Manga sent additional financial support, as did my brother and his wife. Other family members sent donations, and everyone sent prayers. Ian and Rose, since they were both midwives living in the Philippines with us at the time, mostly took turns so that one stayed in Olongapo with their children while the other was on the ground overseeing the disaster response.

RECOVERY EFFORTS

Mercy In Action has remained deeply involved in the ongoing recovery from the super typhoon to this day. Following best-practice guidelines, we kept our acute relief efforts short and, at approximately two months post-disaster, turned our attention to helping local midwives return to their own clinics and birth centers. In the first two years following the disaster, we were able to completely rebuild, refurnish, and restock two birthing facilities on Leyte Island, thanks to grants and generous donations resulting from our fundraising efforts on behalf of the survivors. Mercy In Action also rebuilt a home for Nerissa and her family on the second floor of their birth center building and later added a large classroom to Nerissa's clinic to benefit both patients and local midwives.

Throughout our ongoing disaster response, we have engaged in capacity building. A generous grant from the Center for Disaster Philanthropy enabled us to provide focused and structured capacity building for midwives in the region following the disaster. For a full year after the typhoon, we trained local midwives on best practices in maternity care. Each participant received replacement birth bags to enable them to return to full service as community midwives.

Because of the support we received and the faithful dedication of our local staff, we returned again and again to the disaster zone in the years following the disaster, bringing new classes, birth supplies and equipment, and fresh encouragement each time. Many of the midwives in the area now practice with updated emergency skills they did not have before the typhoon disaster. Having skilled community midwives back in service has become an important part of recovery for this hard-struck region.

Although we rebuilt with no strings attached, Nerissa and Alex decided they wanted to be a permanent part of our team, and made sure her new facility met all the requirements to be a Mercy In Action-supported birth center. In 2021, she and Alex identified another area that had been hard-hit by the typhoon on neighboring Samar Island, where families were still struggling because maternity care was scarce and unaffordable. We were privileged to support the construction of a third birthing facility there, which brings high-quality, free midwifery care to another community struggling to recover.

At the time it hit the Philippines, Super Typhoon Haiyan/Yolanda was the strongest tropical storm ever recorded to make landfall in a populated area, leading to a devastating loss of life, property, and livelihood. Sixteen million people were affected, with approximately 6,000 people killed outright by the massive storm surge that swept through entire towns and villages along the island's coastal region. Besides the immediate death toll, thousands of people were missing, and over 30,000 were injured, with millions homeless and displaced. Untold numbers were buried in mass graves in the chaotic cleanup efforts of these first few months.

I still find it extraordinary that not only were we able to quickly mount an immediate disaster response, but we were also able to help with reconstruction and recovery. In the aftermath, Mercy In Action developed a birth model for maternity care disaster response that we know will work for others facing similar situations.

RELIEF AND DEVELOPMENT

There is a time for relief work, and there is a time for development. Together, they form the foundation of true capacity building, whether in the aftermath of disaster or in places marked by deep and persistent poverty. Relief work meets urgent needs in moments of crisis, but development plants the seeds of resilience. One preserves life in the present, while the other strengthens the ability to survive and thrive into the future.

Lasting transformation occurs when communities are not merely helped, but equipped to do the work themselves. Training midwives, educating families, and building local systems of quality and compassionate healthcare create a legacy far beyond any temporary intervention. In this way, compassion becomes sustainable, and aid becomes empowerment that lasts.

FOR AND AMONG MIDWIVES

Capacity building in midwifery can take two essential forms. There is the work of building capacity *for* midwives, as we offer training, updated practices, and donate essential supplies to strengthen those serving in low-resource settings. And there is the work of building capacity *among* midwives, as local practitioners share skills and wisdom with one another after our trainings and continue to grow as a community, sharing knowledge with each other. Together, these efforts create a foundation that supports safer births, stronger skills among midwives, and lasting change in the places where it is needed most.

I have been talking about our disaster response, but let's switch gears and talk about capacity building in any area of poverty and deprivation. We may not realize how important it is, in capacity building, to reinforce attitudes and skills on both ends of the Safe Labor Spectrum Awareness chart. Everywhere I go, I find that birth providers can too easily fall into doing too little too late or too much too soon. This is dangerous anywhere, but it is especially deadly in areas where health is fragile and emergency care may be lacking. One of our roles in capacity building is to keep coming back to the strong evidence for providing just-right care—the right amount at the right time in the right way.

TOO MUCH AND NOT ENOUGH

When Chevel went into labor, she was admitted to a local midwife-led birth center, one of many in the Philippines, often called lying-in clinics (this one was not affiliated with our organization). A mutual friend accompanied her, who later told me this story. Chevel had no risk factors at the start of labor. Even so, the two midwives caring for her started an intravenous line (IV) and, without Chevel's permission and with no medical indication, added oxytocic drugs to the IV to speed the labor. During the second stage, one midwife suddenly began shoving again and again on the top of Chevel's abdomen, so hard that it rocked the delivery table. At the same time, another midwife cut a large episiotomy, although there were no signs of fetal distress. The midwives never asked for permission for any of this harmful intervention; they simply said they were helping her to give birth. All these procedures are outside the scope of midwifery practice in the Philippines, and should never be done during a normal labor. Yet midwives see these same things done by doctors in the hospitals where they trained, and they imitate what they see, even when practicing outside of a hospital.

Routine fundal pressure and episiotomy are particularly condemned as dangerous practices, yet the harmful behaviors persist in many clinical settings in low- and middle-income countries. The human cost of these practices can be devastating; fundal pushing is linked to fetal brain injury and cerebral palsy in the baby, and placental abruption and uterine rupture in the mother, while episiotomy is responsible for excessive bleeding, infection, pelvic floor damage, and other long-term reproductive complications.

After Chevel's baby was born in this violent fashion, the midwife cut the cord right away and roughly pulled out the placenta, then the baby was taken from the room. This entire birth sequence of events exemplifies what has been called "too much too soon," the inappropriate overuse of medical intervention in a normal laboring mother. Overuse of interventions can and often does cause harm, so it is not surprising that Chevel began to bleed excessively postpartum.

Sadly, this is the point in the story where "too little too late" took over (the inappropriate underuse of intervention when a birth complication occurs). Chevel was given a single medication to control the bleeding, but not the full bundle of hemorrhage care that is universally recommended. The baby had been whisked away five minutes after birth to be weighed, measured, bathed, dressed, and placed in a plastic bed in a separate room. No one thought to help Chevel begin breastfeeding, an activity known to contract the mother's uterus to slow down postpartum bleeding as well as being best practice for a newly born baby.

Though I had seen similar scenes with my own eyes many times over decades in the Philippines, this story was recent and reminded me that entrenched behaviors are hard to change, even after decades of evidence-based recommendations. It reinforced for me that continued efforts to mentor birth practitioners in the balance of "just-right care" are of vital importance to good outcomes everywhere. Anyone wanting to improve maternity care could go almost anywhere in the world and make a difference simply by teaching how to better support natural birth when it is working and how to respond appropriately when complications arise. If we can get this balance right, we can help mothers and babies survive and thrive. That is why capacity building for and among midwives is essential to building a world where it is safe to give birth.

There is a saying in leadership circles that your vision should fit on a T-shirt. Our visionary motto is not complicated, and it is literally on the back of our T-shirts: "Safe Motherhood and Newborn Survival, One Good Birth at a Time." This short saying expresses the profound yet simple goal of all our efforts, encompassing our commitment to standard best practices clinically and in community health education. Safe birth and good birth must go together.

Capacity building does not need to focus only on the delivery room. Childbirth education as one small part of community development is so important. Let's switch gears again and look at some examples of using outreach for capacity building that leans into a celebratory atmosphere to improve maternity outcomes. We are limited only by our imaginations in how we can improve the underlying culture around birth, in big ways and in small ways.

MAKE IT A CELEBRATION

Infusing a joyful spirit into maternity care is a powerful way to cement learning while building a strong sense of community and belonging. I have midwife friends and former students around the world who are especially gifted at turning learning into fun. In Manila, I have watched Jeri and her daughter, Deb, lead their team of midwives in hosting learning-through-games childbirth classes, filled with laughter and lively participation. They make every mother feel valued and infuse their childbirth education with principles of community development and empowerment. In Madagascar, Alissa and Rota and their team of midwives have created a model of participatory learning that engages the mothers and holds their interest long after giving birth. They have mothers enroll in a program they commit to for the entirety of the pregnancy and for six months after. Both centers host large, festive graduation ceremonies to honor mothers and fathers who complete their full course of childbirth and parenting teachings.

What would it look like if we all started looking for an excuse to throw a party as part of our care package? What if we planned festive gatherings that celebrate the hard work it takes to grow a healthy baby and raise a thriving family? In communities burdened by poverty and stress, shared joy can become a surprising engine for capacity building. In two very different places, I have seen what happens when generosity takes the shape of a people-powered celebration.

FAITH-BASED STREET PARTY

My dear friends Ernie and Linda Neria were preparing to start a church plant in a hardscrabble rural town in New Mexico that sits near the borderlands of Texas and Mexico. The Neria family is Mexican American, with Native American roots, a heritage that naturally shaped how they lived and served in a region where Spanish is widely spoken and cultural ties run deep. Together with their four sons, they were committed to walking alongside their neighbors and serving their community in the name of Christ. I had the joy of briefly serving alongside them during the years we lived on the Mexican border and traveled back and forth to the Philippines.

From the start of this new venture, the Neria family had dreamed of a church based on outreach that met real needs in the community. This included plans for a food bank, since most families in the region lived below the poverty line. I was honored to come alongside them in a small way as they pursued their vision of a countercultural faith community that would welcome everyone and meet both spiritual and practical needs. In planning for this, I wondered what might happen if we combined free healthcare with the free food, offering dignified compassion to meet a felt need among young families. Concerned as we were with reaching the most vulnerable populations, and knowing that any degree of malnutrition during pregnancy and the early years can be permanently damaging to the child, we added prenatal care and early childhood health screenings to the food bank outreach for the season I worked with them.

Food bank nights in Chaparral became an event that felt more like a fiesta than charity. Rather organically, an evening street party evolved. Being a musical family, Ernie and one or two of his boys brought their guitars and put on a mini concert each week from the bed of a parked truck on the street. Crates of fresh vegetables and fruits were offered to anyone who came by. My team of midwives provided free pregnancy checkups in a building on-site, and taught parents how to track the weight and developmental milestones of their babies and young children. Between songs, we gave short health teachings in English and Spanish, often tying the health message to a spiritual concept. Prayer was on the menu, often requested and freely given, but we were careful to make sure people knew it was not a requirement for receiving healthcare. The healthcare was given freely, like the food, without any strings attached.

It wasn't a complex system, nor was it comprehensive healthcare, but it started making a difference. Women who had previously been shut out of maternity care due to a lack of ability to pay were now receiving prenatal exams early in their pregnancies. Parents brought their children to us to be weighed and assessed because they could visit our food bank at night, while the health center in their community closed before they got off work. Imagine what the outcome might be if every church food pantry could turn into a street party where maternal and child healthcare and education were delivered alongside food distribution?

PHILIPPINES BUNTIS PARTY

At our Mercy In Action sponsored birth centers in the Philippines, Nerissa envisioned and launched a creative gathering to honor and support pregnant women (*buntis*) in the disaster-stricken communities surrounding her birth centers. She was first inspired by a commercial event held in large Philippine cities called a Buntis Congress, which primarily targets middle- and upper-class women and is held in big urban shopping malls. Nerissa transformed that idea by moving it from malls to rural villages and shifting the focus from those with resources to those with the greatest need. She reshaped it into something uniquely generous in spirit by centering each gathering on the sharing of knowledge, food, and belonging.

Many women are living in dire circumstances when they first find their way to Mercy In Action through a Buntis Party. They often tell us that when they first heard rumors about these gatherings coming to their community, they thought it must be too good to be true, and yet it became their first doorway into maternity care.

PLANNING AND EXECUTION

Mercy In Action's Buntis Parties are carefully planned several times each year on each of the three islands where we primarily serve, with the venue rotating among underserved areas. The midwives announce the upcoming Buntis Party through social media, posters, and word of mouth. They coordinate with barangay health workers and local officials, who are then given a platform at the Buntis Party to share what services the local health center offers.

On the day of the event, everyone is ushered into a large space, often a covered basketball court or large courtyard. Like most events in the Philippines, the program begins with a brief prayer, followed by a word of greeting from a local government official. After these formalities, the heart of the day begins: teaching about the importance of the first 1,000 days of life, including a safe and respectful birth. The attendees learn that their children's long-term health begins during the earliest days of pregnancy, and there is much they can do to move the odds in their favor of having a healthy baby.

Learning games are often held, and prizes are given. Most of the prizes are practical items a family can use to stay healthy, such as mosquito nets, water containers, and other household goods. Each buntis goes home with a gift bag containing vitamins and a small clothing item for her newborn. Finally, a nourishing meal is served to all in attendance, including any older children or family members who came with the mother. Our midwives are wonderful at hosting these parties with exuberance, and a sense of playful fun keeps the mood high throughout.

For many participants, the greatest gift is the invitation to start prenatal care, free of charge, that very day. Because of our Open Access model, the ticket in the door to our birth center is pregnancy, not money. No woman is pressured to leave her current provider if she has one, but many women who attend have not yet had any prenatal care. Every woman is offered a safe, respectful delivery at no charge, with the promise that we will also follow her baby's growth and development for two full years after birth with monthly home visits.

As you can imagine, the community looks on these gatherings as more than parties. They are a deep act of hospitality, creativity, and generosity. They are a bridge to prenatal care, and a living witness to the pathway created by ICI, which calls for collaboration between government and private providers. For many mothers, the Buntis Party is the first time anyone has clearly communicated that she and her baby deserve the very best care possible.

INVESTMENT IN EDUCATION AS CAPACITY BUILDING

No matter how generous we hope to be, we cannot share what we do not have. We must remain committed to lifelong learning and freely pass along new knowledge to those who need it. That may be someone pregnant in your neighborhood, a health professional, or a student. It may be a neighbor right next door, or perhaps you may travel across the world to offer help to a stranger. By gaining knowledge and sharing it, we become a blessing to future generations of parents and midwives on the front lines of survival in maternal and child health. Knowledge becomes generosity when we pass it on.

GENEROSITY IN TRAINING

Through Mercy In Action seminars and workshops, we have for decades given away continuing education to national midwives in my adopted country, the Philippines. Yet I have long dreamed of the opportunity to make a deeper impact on primary midwifery education there, the way we do in the USA through the Mercy In Action College of Midwifery. It was Nerissa, visionary that she is, who first spotted an opportunity to become a clinical preceptor at her alma mater. Nerissa has since contracted with two other local midwifery colleges to provide a clinical learning site where next-generation midwives have a rare chance to witness evidence-based midwifery practiced in accordance with the universally recommended midwifery model of care.

Led exclusively by local Filipina midwives, Nerissa's birth center is a teaching site where students learn what it truly means to practice safe and respectful maternity care with excellence. They are setting a powerful example for their community and the entire country of the Philippines by doing the hard work of maintaining facility site status with the International Childbirth Initiative (ICI): 12 Steps to Safe and Respectful MotherBaby-Family Maternity Care.

It is no small thing to be trained in such a place. As I noted in an earlier chapter, the International Childbirth Initiative is concerned with both baby-friendly and mother-friendly facility care. Its steps were agreed upon by the International Confederation of Midwives, the International Federation of Gynecology and Obstetrics, and the International Pediatric Association, representing the professions most directly involved in childbirth. As implementing sites of the ICI, our birth centers have become ideal training environments. They help form the next generation of midwives in the Philippines by showing, day after day, that birth can be both safer and more respectful than most students have ever experienced. Our midwifery model of care serves as both the example and the goal.

TRAINING ALLIES TO PROMOTE HEALTH

Generous investment in education is not limited to midwives. The work of safe motherhood and child survival is strengthened every time we equip doulas, childbirth educators, natural birth advocates, young people interested in global health, and anyone else who is willing to learn and effect change in their own communities. When we share what we know with openness and intention, we multiply the impact into places we may never stand ourselves. Teaching others to teach is one of the most powerful forms of service. Maternal and child health trainers become part of a much larger movement to protect mothers and babies. Generosity in education plants seeds that grow far beyond our sight, and often far beyond our lifetime.

Every pregnant woman, and every partner or family member who supports her, deserves to know how to grow a healthy baby, give birth safely, and care for that child in the very best way. Whether you are a birth worker or a parent, a teacher, a neighbor, a friend, or simply someone who cares, you can learn the most powerful facts for life and pass them along to those who need them. Pregnancy education needs to reach the only person who can directly influence the growing baby during the first 280 days of the first 1,000 days of life, and that is the mother carrying the child within her womb. When we teach her well and surround her with a community that supports her, we give both mother and baby a stronger beginning and a better chance to survive and thrive. This is all part of our vision and strategy for better birth outcomes.

YOUTH MERCY TEAM

One of the most unconventional yet meaningful teaching projects I ever undertook grew out of my decade serving as the mission pastor at a church on the US-Mexico border. When my sons were teenagers, I formed a group of high-school- and college-age kids that we came to call the Youth Mercy Team. About twenty teens from the church met with me every Sunday afternoon to learn healthcare ministry. Together, we worked our way through the subjects in UNICEF's *Facts for Life* book, and they learned how to teach basic health lessons to pregnant mothers and parents. During this time, I tried to instill in them a heart for marginalized people, and they didn't have far to look to see the needs all around us. They came to understand the struggles of families living in poverty with limited access to care and resources. They internalized the belief that service begins with them, and they stepped into the role with passion and compassion, surprising those accustomed to looking down on teenagers.

All summer long, these kids gave up one day a week to serve at our clinic in Mexico, working side by side with our midwives and pediatrician. They mastered vital signs and injections while assisting our pediatrician, and shadowed our midwives to learn the basics of prenatal care and newborn exams. They put on skits and puppet shows each week to demonstrate the health messages they had learned, using drama, theater, music, and art to convey facts for life.

Summers were hot in our northern Mexico climate, but winters brought freezing weather for months. It was all too common to hear of babies freezing to death on cold winter nights in the communities we served. So every autumn, my Youth Mercy Team, boys and girls alike, began crocheting thick baby blankets to give away. We held a Saint Martinmas Day outreach to distribute the blankets to families with small children each November 11 in commemoration of Martin of Tours's example of generosity to the poor. As winter approached, they spent Saturdays working beside Scott and me and other adults from our church, winterizing houses in the desert on the edge of Juarez, where people built tiny homes with cardboard boxes. At Christmastime, we wrapped and delivered gifts of household items and food to families struggling to survive in their desperately poor colonias. The Youth Mercy Team rose to these occasions for service with sincerity and courage, and they grew into capable helpers who offered meaningful support to the families we cared for. By their own testimonies, many were shaped for life by what they experienced during that season.

Randy Ponzio was one such young man who joined my Youth Mercy Team. I can still see him playing with children in Mexico while weighing and measuring them, making up silly songs to teach them health messages. He seemed drawn to the children who had been overlooked, the ones whose unwashed faces and torn, rumpled clothes showed how much neglect they had experienced in their young lives. Kids starved for affection found a friend in Randy, and he lifted them without hesitation, sometimes carrying two or three on his back, giving them his full attention as if they mattered more than anything else in the world.

Randy became an unlikely ambassador for maternal and child health. A bold proponent of breastfeeding after he found out how much it mattered to a child's future health and brain development, he was always extolling its value in all his teaching and loudly declared that mothers were "dope for breastfeeding" whenever he saw one nursing her baby in our waiting room. He was our secret weapon because of his huge heart for suffering people combined with his comic timing in presenting health messages.

One Christmas season, I showed the movie *The Fourth Wise Man* to a group of our young leaders. It is based on the classic by Henry van Dyke, *The Story of the Other Wise Man*, a fictional tale set in biblical times. The story relates the misadventures of a wise man who never makes it to Bethlehem, as he keeps getting waylaid by the needs of people along the way. He searches his entire life for the Christ child, but although he never finds Jesus, he finds lots of poor people to serve. In the end, as he lies dying, he hears the voice of Christ tell him, "Whatsoever you have done to the least of these my brothers, you have done to me." It is admittedly a moving scene, but none of us anticipated its effect on Randy. As the credits rolled, we heard a deep groaning rise into sobs, and when the lights came up we saw him face down on the floor, weeping. I remember thinking with awe that Randy was receiving that most precious and rare gift, a heart broken for the things that break the heart of God, and he was not ashamed to fully embrace the pain of that.

Later, Randy and his new wife joined our team in the Philippines. I was privileged to midwife the birth of their first child, witnessing Randy become a father who loved his own children with the same enthusiasm he lavished on other people's children. Sadly, Randy died far too young, a crushing loss for his family and for all of us who had the privilege of knowing him. Yet his legacy lives on in the stories we still tell and in the lives he touched. It was a joy to witness that season when young hearts like Randy's were being shaped for a lifetime of mercy through their brief foray into healthcare learning and service.

TRAIN THE TRAINER

Mercy In Action leaders have an ongoing desire to live out a model that truly works in global maternal and newborn health. We are involved in providing maternity care and training others to do the same, and we are trying our hardest to do so in a way that is culturally appropriate.

We recognize that, in many ways, midwifery provided by expatriates is problematic, and new paradigms are sorely needed. It has been noted that when well-meaning healthcare workers return home at the end of their stint with nothing sustainable left behind, it sometimes leaves the host country's midwives, doctors, nurses and community health workers feeling more disempowered.

Through Mercy In Action we now propose a new model based on the "train the trainer" concept. Rather than traveling to other countries simply to "catch babies" or to gain experience, midwives are invited into the more valuable and sustainable work of capacity building in communities that struggle to provide quality maternity care under difficult conditions. Midwives from wealthier nations partner with midwives in developing countries to train local leaders in updated, evidence-based best practices. This approach helps avoid unhealthy power differentials and builds lasting local strength.

One effective way to do this is by sharing the curricula of Helping Mothers and Babies Survive courses. In our train-the-trainer workshops, we encourage participants to purchase and bring the Laerdal Global Health interactive training dolls and uterus models known as MamaNatalie and NeoNatalie with them when they go to low-resource countries. These tools are then left behind for the permanent use of local midwives, strengthening training capacity long after volunteers have returned home.

Another strategy is to equip and empower local birth practitioners in the visited country to follow the International Childbirth Initiative (ICI). Since the twelve steps emphasize natural childbirth and breastfeeding as well as emergency-response skills, community midwives become safer and better prepared to serve pregnant women.

Through this strategy we hope to redirect the current flow of international volunteers into a movement that changes the paradigm. Rather than focusing primarily on the experience gained by visiting midwives, this model emphasizes what is left behind. It builds lasting local capacity, strengthens midwifery, and improves birth outcomes for mothers and babies around the world. And the great thing is, this can be taught to midwives by anyone who is trained, no need to be a midwife yourself.

While the world has seen a reduction in maternal and infant mortality in the past decade, the numbers are still unacceptably high and the suffering largely preventable. Providers of maternity care in low-resource countries lack supplies, training, and encouragement in their fight to save the lives of these mothers and newborns in their care. Mercy In Action exists to change that situation to the best of our ability, and we invite you to join us in this vision. We want to teach the train-the-trainer model so we can multiply the good work midwives do on a global scale, for better outcomes everywhere we visit, live, work, or volunteer!

SHARE OUTCOME STATISTICS

Whatever you do in midwifery practice or education, share your outcomes. An incredibly important part of Mercy in Action's visionary strategy is keeping careful track of statistics on the midwifery care we provide. We keep detailed records on all our births. Data helps us understand what is happening in our care and guides us toward improvement. Starting when I was in Alaska as a twenty-something midwife, I have shared my year-end statistics with doctors in my community. They need to know, and it is a way to keep the lines of communication open and impress them with how many babies are being born outside of hospitals without problems, since the only ones they see are transfers for complications.

Over the years, thanks to Scott's early vision for capturing our birth data, we have published our Philippine outcomes for each of the thousands of births at our Mercy In Action-sponsored birth centers. Filipina midwives record the data in real time, we pay a local computer expert, Mark Ian, to collect and store the data, and Nicole, our brilliant and generous volunteer researcher, keeps us up-to-date by sorting and categorizing the usable data every few years. In this way, we can see where our outcomes remain strong and where we have room to improve.

GIVING KNOWLEDGE AWAY IN THE COMMUNITY

When I worked as a young midwife in Alaska, first in private practice and later as the founder of a nonprofit, I found it a joy to share knowledge freely with my communities, offering free pre-pregnancy and early-pregnancy health education as a practical expression of care and concern for everyone. We also offered more traditional childbirth preparation in our birth center; however, it was these free early classes that helped families get a solid start on understanding how to grow a healthy baby from the very beginning, with clear, evidence-based guidance. It was a "first 1,000 days" program before I even knew the phrase!

Today, in the Philippines, our midwives freely share knowledge about childbirth in women's prisons, area hospitals and health centers, in squatter areas, and at the local garbage dump. Most parents we serve live in varying levels of poverty and have limited access to information. Sometimes their elders may be giving them harmful, outdated advice, such as encouraging bottle-feeding or dehydrating a baby who has diarrhea. So our non-judgemental community teaching sessions become an open door to life-saving knowledge for entire communities across generations, helping change outcomes far into the future.

Another educational opportunity for capacity building in our communities is the clinic waiting room, where vital knowledge is shared every day while patients wait for their prenatal or postpartum exam. Besides the live teachings, beautiful pre-recorded audio-visual lessons play on the tv screen, covering topics related to the important first 1,000 days, including early brain development, nutrition during pregnancy, newborn care, and the importance of breastfeeding. These teachings are in the local language of each island where we have a birth center. Our waiting rooms provide a steady flow of information that parents and the family members who join them can absorb at their own pace. It is a simple system that reaches thousands of families each year and reflects our conviction that informed parents, relatives, and friends of the family are powerful partners in improving birth outcomes.

INNOVATIONS IN HEALTH EDUCATION DELIVERY

When we innovate, we think outside the box. This can allow us to make all kinds of positive changes possible through health education delivery. As the message of the book *Facts for Life* reminds us, there are basic topics every person has a right to know. We can grow more creative and more strategic in our vision for bringing these lifesaving facts into our communities and into the consciousness of those who stand to benefit most from them. Let's commit to sharing ideas, techniques, wisdom, and ongoing knowledge acquisition with each other and keep on growing together!

A SHINING EXAMPLE

During her third year as a student at our Mercy In Action College of Midwifery, Paula Marti traveled to the Philippines to take part in an international event we held at our clinic locations. Paula arrived in the islands eager to learn and witness our midwifery model in action, and she quickly absorbed both the practical side of our model and the heart behind our mission work. After completing the Helping Mothers and Babies Survive courses as a student learner, she turned around the next day and taught the local Filipina midwives, earning her Master Trainer status and preparing her for a future far beyond what she may have imagined at the time.

Fast forward two years. Within two months of graduating with her midwifery degree, Paula was standing in an open village setting in

Uganda, Africa, training local midwives on lifesaving techniques. I remember the photo she sent me of that moment, where surrounded by a small circle of attentive women, she taught with calm confidence in the heat of the day. Even in the picture I could see the transformation that had taken place in Paula. She had moved from student to teacher, from one who learned under supervision to one who now leads, teaches, and equips others to save lives. She told me this week that she had begun raising funds to help build a birth center in this village in Uganda. I was pleased but not surprised.

Paula's journey is a powerful reflection of the formation we hope to cultivate in our students, whether they serve in America or abroad after graduation. It is not only about clinical skill and knowledge. It is just as much about courage, humility, and a willingness to step forward when called, even into unfamiliar places, for the sake of mothers and babies.

THE WEIGHT WE CARRY

Although we have had great success overall in our global programs and disaster responses, not all stories end well. When we set out to help in desperate situations of poverty or disaster, we need to remember that life is not ultimately something we control. While it is rare for us to lose a life under our care, this past Christmas season, I experienced the heartbreak of attending two wakes for small babies who we had been following in our First 1,000 Days program in the Philippines.

The first wake was for little Ren. We had just been talking about how well he was doing on his growth chart at almost two years old, when one day, while playing, his breathing suddenly became labored, and on the frantic ride to the hospital, he died in his mother's arms.

I drove to visit his wake in the rain, navigating narrow streets in a very poor community near the ocean. I stood wet and soggy beneath a torn tarp and peered into his small, open casket with my arm around his mother, who was still a teenager herself. I held her and prayed over her there in the muddy, makeshift shelter, with neighbors gambling at a card table beside the casket. The gambling may seem strange to an outsider, but it is a tradition and the way poor families get money to pay the funeral home to bury their loved one.

Since autopsy is not common here, we are left not knowing why Ren died so suddenly. He had been visited every month and seemed healthy, but now he was gone, and there was nothing left to do except comfort his grieving family. The rain felt right, like tears from heaven.

The second death came only a week later, to a baby we had never even met. Algie's mom had her prenatal care with us but went to the local hospital for birth and ended up with a cesarean delivery. Whisked away right after he was born, baby Algie's parents were never allowed to see him, and no one explained why he was in the NICU. Then one day, two weeks after his birth, they were told their baby was being transferred to another hospital an hour away for immediate surgery. A kind doctor at the second hospital explained about an internal blockage, and for the first time his parents were allowed to hold him. Sadly, while surgery was being arranged, his intestines ruptured, and little Algie died. His mother and father watched helplessly and wept.

For the second time in eight days, our clinic staff and I took ourselves off to a wake, this time at the local landfill, where his family lived because they scavenged through garbage for a living. This wake was also not a nice place to visit. Stepping over reeking trash, I felt even more heartbroken by the conditions when I saw that the ground beneath my feet was crawling with maggots. We made our way over obstacles to climb a small hill, and at the top, duck down a narrow alley to the small room where Algie lay. There we offered what small comfort we could, gathering around the tiny open coffin to pay our respects and cry with the mother as she told us intimate details of his short life. Again, after months of prenatal care and follow-up visits to the hospital, there was nothing left to do but bear witness to the family's pain.

These are the times it is hard to remember we are making a difference in the big picture. Yet these stories are part of the reality of this work, too, and there is an important concept here: When we cannot save a life, comfort becomes the ministry. The ministry of presence is showing up when you have nothing left to give. Even on a muddy street and on a garbage dumpsite—perhaps especially in such places—just showing up is holy. By entering these sacred spaces where grief is raw, we honor the lives that were here so briefly, and we affirm that the life lost was precious. Our presence shows the grieving family that they are not alone in their sorrow.

UNEVEN DISTRIBUTION

In the Philippines where I live, I have heard this saying: "A pregnant woman has one foot in the grave." The liminal space surrounding the time of childbirth is felt in many low-resource countries, where women may say goodbye to their older children when labor starts.

Maternal death, though much rarer than child death, is still treacherously high, on average a hundred times higher in low-resource countries than in richer nations. Globally, the leading causes of maternal death remain bleeding, infections, obstructed labor, and eclampsia. These conditions and their sequela account for the largest share of maternal loss around the world. What makes this reality especially painful is that all these conditions are preventable and treatable when timely and appropriate care is available. Women are not dying because solutions are unknown. They are dying because access to those solutions remains unevenly distributed and too often out of reach for those who can never earn enough to pay for them.

Part of the problem is a worldwide shortage of midwives. According to the International Confederation of Midwives' statement released in 2025, the world needs at least one million more midwives to meet the needs. Having a midwife or other skilled health worker at every delivery is a major key to improving outcomes, and WHO officials wrote on their website that "Investing in human capital such as midwives for childbirth is the wisest investment that we make, to ensure sustainability, ownership, fulfillment, and consistently high results."

This reminds us once again that not everyone needs to be boots on the ground. Not everyone needs to become a midwife themselves to fight this battle. If you make donations to works like ours, you too are making the "wisest investment" in what will pay the highest dividends in the end.

SUSTAINING EXCELLENCE

One of the greatest dangers in any organization is not failure, but drift. The very practices that once defined compassionate, excellent care can slowly begin to erode under the pressure of increasing demands, staff shortages, and simple human exhaustion. In the Philippine birth centers that we support, anywhere from ten to fifty babies are born every month. The global shortage of midwives I have been discussing in this book is not theoretical to us; we live within this reality every day.

Last year, we realized that one important part of our care model had slipped. Home visits after birth for postpartum care in the first week, which we consider essential, were becoming inconsistent. As the midwives worked hard and made sacrifices to meet the overwhelming needs, they began asking mothers to return to the birth center outpatient clinic for follow-up care in the first weeks after birth. But when we carefully examined our records, we found that less than half of the mothers returned for postpartum care.

When this gap came to our attention, we sought to address it collectively alongside our national midwife leaders. Excellence cannot be sustained through criticism or blame but through honest evaluation, humility, creativity, and a willingness to solve problems together. We discussed practical solutions with the leaders and eventually decided to hire and train nurses specifically to assist with postpartum home visits, under the supervision of the licensed midwives. This adjustment helped restore an important layer of care that families needed and deserved, even amid a severe midwife shortage.

As we looked more closely at the problem, we realized the gap was larger than one birth center. As we closely examined the ICI materials to identify areas of accountability, to our surprise, we found that the guidance there was also lacking. We researched WHO guidance on postpartum care (amount and timing of visits), and we shared it with our birth center leaders. During a recent ICI advisory committee meeting, we mentioned the need to stress postpartum care by referring to WHO guidance on this subject. It became clear that this was an area needing stronger emphasis, clearer guidance, and renewed attention in a broader sense.

Experiences like this remind me that quality control is never a finished task. Good systems do not sustain themselves automatically. Left unattended, even meaningful practices can slowly disappear beneath the weight of urgent demands. Even strong cultures require continual attention, evaluation, and course correction.

LOOK FOR THE HELPERS

Fred Rogers, the beloved American television personality and Presbyterian minister, recounted how as a young boy he was sometimes frightened by disasters he saw on the news. Fred Rogers recalled that his mother would say, "Always look for the helpers. There will always be helpers."

Capacity building is helping. And as I end this chapter, I want to make the observation that scientific research increasingly shows that it is in helping and serving that we ourselves become most satisfied with our own lives. It seems we may be wired, as human beings, to feel happiest when we are helping others.

A few of you reading this will decide to help others by crossing borders to share your skills and resources. Many others can support charitable midwifery work by donating, advocating, and supporting midwives working in low-resource areas. In every season of my life, I have seen that generosity is a way of life that transforms both the giver and the receiver, and generosity in maternity care always improves outcomes. It only takes asking, "What can I do to help?"

PAUSE FOR REFLECTION

In what ways do you desire to be more generous in your efforts to improve maternity care? Are you interested in considering the principles of leading from behind? Who do you know that is providing capacity building to midwives in situations of poverty or disaster, and what can you learn from that person's example?

11
ACTION FOR IMPACT

When you learn, teach. When you get, give.

— MAYA ANGELOU

GENEROSITY IS, AT ITS CORE, A POSTURE OF THE HEART. SO WHEN WE question where to focus our energy, it is wise to begin not with ways to improve our skills or strategies, though that is important, but with the condition of our hearts. Knowledge can be updated, and skills can be practiced, but ultimately it is our heart attitudes that shape how we engage with the world and how we show up in our care for others.

If our hearts are open, humble, and generous, our interactions will be deeper and more rewarding, our strategy will be more focused on achieving positive outcomes for those we serve, and our service will be more faithful. It is from a place of rooted purpose that we can step forward into the future with a more generous way of being in the world.

If, on the other hand, we find that our hearts have grown hurried, weary, and self-protective, it may be time to renew ourselves, lest we fall short of giving the love and care that those we serve truly need and deserve during pregnancy, birth, and beyond.

I want to invite you to prepare inwardly first, because everything else flows from the heart. The journey always begins within, and everyone makes new choices daily, whether they choose to do the same old things or decide to be lifelong learners, open to new creative possibilities.

In this chapter I will describe the midwifery and maternal and child health learning opportunities my organization offers. From there, I will point you toward resources that have helped me stay current as I continue to grow professionally and spiritually in this work. Finally, I will challenge you to create a plan going forward after finishing this book, a roadmap to keep growing and sharing knowledge for your lifetime. Whether or not we are midwives, we can all work to "midwife mercy" in the lives of others through creative, life-changing strategies.

THE JOURNEY OF LIFELONG LEARNING

We can only give good gifts to others if we attend to our own ongoing growth and development. It begins with a commitment to lifelong learning and to cultivating a growth mindset. This dedication to continued learning and growing is followed by a responsibility to generously share the knowledge and wisdom gained. Within the field of maternal and child health, a culture of sharing knowledge enriches both the giver and the receiver, and better birth outcomes are bound to follow.

Lifelong learning is essential for any midwife who hopes to serve with excellence and integrity. Our work keeps changing as new research develops and best practices evolve. When we stay current through continuing education or the pursuit of higher degrees, we strengthen our clinical judgment, deepen our confidence, and widen our understanding of the people and communities we serve. Ongoing study and reflection help us grow in knowledge and wisdom, and they prepare us for the complex challenges of this calling.

Midwives are teachers in the community, offering wisdom to pregnant families. When we pass on what we know, freely and respectfully, we multiply the impact of our learning. A midwife who teaches a parent how best to prepare for birth, or who guides a student apprentice with patience, extends the reach of every lesson she has carried along the way. Our hearts must be fully engaged if learning and sharing knowledge are to be deeply valued and freely given within a shared community.

GROWTH MINDSET

I have found over and over that the best midwives, teachers, and leaders I know have a growth mindset. Psychologist Carol Dweck describes a growth mindset as the belief that our abilities and understanding can be developed through effort, learning, and experience. A fixed mindset, by contrast, assumes that what we know and who we are professionally are largely set, leaving little room for growth or improvement.

As midwives and those who support midwives, we should intentionally choose a growth mindset, remaining open, curious, and committed to learning for the sake of those we serve. To be a responsible midwife is to walk a path of learning that never truly ends; learning definitely does not stop with graduation from midwifery school. Our calling asks us to remain open to new ways of doing things, even after we feel experienced and sure of ourselves. If we cultivate this habit now, embracing a growth mindset becomes a way of life.

Great midwives, like top achievers in any profession, never stop learning, though the journey will look a bit different for everyone. Midwives with a growth mindset will find something to learn from in every situation, whether formal or informal. They remain open to the lessons that come through experience, through the people they interact with, and through the mistakes that teach us more than success ever could.

There is no finish line in the long marathon of learning about maternal and child health, no moment when we arrive at the sum total of all wisdom. This work calls us to remain humble, attentive, and willing to keep growing in understanding over time. If we hope to serve families well, we must stay engaged with evidence-based practice, follow new research, and be willing to integrate new insights with experience. Some of you may eventually contribute your own well-designed studies, adding to the growing body of knowledge that strengthens midwifery and improves birth outcomes for future generations.

AFTER GRADUATION

I encourage every graduate of our midwifery college to begin their career with one simple commitment: Invest in your continuing education. Budget for books. Use the library. Subscribe to online biomedical and health science research databases. Join your state and national midwifery organizations. Take advantage of online courses and webinars. Engage in current research and get involved in research projects as you are able. Stay curious. Keep asking questions. Never stop learning.

By being generous with yourself and investing in your own education throughout your lifetime, you will set yourself up to be a great midwife. If you feel called to pursue graduate degrees after finishing midwifery school, keep an open mind about how that might look for you. It is always a privilege for our college and diploma staff to write letters of recommendation for graduates of Mercy In Action's educational programs who are applying to pursue various postgraduate degrees. Some of our graduates have gone on to earn degrees in related healthcare fields, such as public health, maternal health systems, nursing, and medicine. Some have expanded their circle of study to include fields that complement their midwifery work, such as business, leadership, anthropology, sociology, counseling, and ministry, to name a few.

All this is to say, do everything you can to keep learning for your entire lifetime, whether it is formal education or informal. Midwifery is both a service vocation and a creative space, and every step of learning strengthens the care we offer. Our own personal growth is what shapes the way we practice, the way we lead, and the way we walk out the sacred purpose of this calling in midwifery.

GLOBAL TRAINING STANDARDS

Globally, there are two major pathways to becoming a midwife: one through nursing first and then midwifery education, and one through direct-entry midwifery training without prior nursing. Direct-entry pathways are the most common in many regions of the world, while nurse-midwifery remains prominent in others. (Fun fact: the University of the Philippines uses a unique "ladderized" curriculum in which those hoping to become nurses are trained as midwives first.) One pathway to midwifery is not superior to the other; they are simply different.

It is important to be aware that more and more countries are requiring a minimum of a bachelor of science degree for midwives, and in most places globally, midwifery schools must be accredited to ensure the highest standards. If you are exploring midwifery training for yourself, or advising someone who is preparing to begin, choosing a midwifery school that offers an accredited bachelor's degree can greatly expand future options for where you may live and serve. An accredited midwifery school can also provide the most well-rounded education and has the most robust student protections in place. It is hard to know where your path will lead or where you may be called in the years ahead, so preparing now for flexibility and mobility keeps doors open later.

AN EVOLVING MODEL

When our Mercy In Action model was shared in Robbie Davis-Floyd's seminal book *Birth Models That Work* in 2009, our detailed statistics showed that a midwife-led clinic in a low-resource setting could provide quality care. The model I described in that book included foreign students working alongside national midwives to provide care. While we had good outcomes and closely supervised all students, a few things have changed since then. We now feel that the tenets of cultural competency and respectful and ethical maternity care dictate that only those who fluently speak the patient's heart language should conduct deliveries and other clinical care. Around the time we were deciding that, representatives of the Philippines' Professional Regulation Commission (PRC) came around and made it clear to us that it was not legal to host foreign midwifery students in the Philippines without a PRC license, which they seem to grant solely to their own Filipina midwifery college students. Together, those were two good reasons to close our foreign midwife training program and pivot to focus on educating the next generation of Filipino midwives within the country.

Our new approach is to advocate for midwives to be trained initially in their own country, where they can fully communicate with patients and clients while learning midwifery skills under licensed preceptors. Only after they no longer need anything from patients and clients, but instead have something valuable to give, should they serve as a midwife outside their own country. Within this framework of cultural humility and respect, advocated by many leaders in healthcare training worldwide, the conventional wisdom is to obtain pre-service midwifery training in your own country and culture before pursuing advanced training to serve internationally. With all this in mind, we created a wonderful alternative—we now offer anyone interested in international midwifery or maternal and child health a place in our postgraduate diploma program, which I will describe later in this chapter.

MERCY IN ACTION LEARNING OPPORTUNITIES

Mercy In Action is more committed than ever to addressing the world's maternal and child healthcare needs, and we have created a rich mix of educational programs to serve learners globally. Apart from our USA-based midwifery college, our many continuing education offerings are open to residents of every country in the world, and include online courses, workshops, seminars, and our diploma program. We have scholars taking our classes from dozens of countries around the world—midwives, doulas, childbirth educators, nurses, doctors, health advocates, philanthropists, and donors. In fact, we have scholars on every continent except Antarctica!

We will start by looking at the initial midwifery training Mercy In Action offers, designed to instill midwifery vision, mission, heart, and evidence-based strategy in the next generation of midwives. We will then move on to our in-service continuing education for practicing midwives and other birth workers. These educational programs are a big part of how we are shaping better outcomes in birth, everywhere in the world.

MERCY IN ACTION COLLEGE OF MIDWIFERY BACHELOR OF SCIENCE DEGREE

While our accredited college is only in the USA, our graduates are impacting the world. All midwife schools teach the basics, but our program is also focused on building the character of a midwife to improve birth outcomes. Global in focus, the Mercy In Action College of Midwifery prepares midwives to be compassionate and responsible global citizens, developing excellence in midwifery knowledge, skills, and attitudes that positively impact the ability of mothers and babies to survive and thrive anywhere in the world.

Our college is a four-year, degree-granting, community-based distance program, accredited by the Midwifery Education Accreditation Council (MEAC) in the USA. The curriculum is designed as a four-year program but can be completed in as little as three years or as long as six, whichever fits the student's situation. The course prepares students to meet the criteria for midwifery training set in part by the International Confederation of Midwives.

Pre-service learning is everything a midwife studies before beginning practice. It includes the formal academic education, supervised clinical experience, and foundational skills required to enter the profession. These are the years when a student midwife learns the basics, asks many questions, and is always carefully supervised clinically while building the competencies needed for safe care. Pre-service learning prepares a midwife to begin.

I have spent years serving learners at every point of this long journey, from the first inkling of a calling right through graduation and passing the board exams to be licensed as a midwife. None of it is easy, but it is doable, and often transformational, for the majority of people who set out on the journey of becoming a midwife.

Research your options carefully when deciding on a midwifery school to attend. There are big differences in program philosophy and student support, as well as length, structure, whether it is degree-granting versus certificate or diploma, and successful graduation rates. Often the best way to learn what you really want to know is by talking to students who have graduated or are currently enrolled. Schools should be willing to give you some names and contact information for alumni who are willing to talk to you and answer your questions.

Through it all, remember that despite the barriers that may arise along the way, such as possible issues of time, money, stress, self-doubt, and lack of family support, most graduates will tell you it is worth it to become a midwife, with all the rights and responsibilities that title entails. Getting a solid educational foundation as a midwife is a step toward the changed outcomes in maternal and newborn survival that we wish for and dream of. Be willing to invest.

GRAND CHALLENGE SCHOLARSHIPS

Since the very beginning of my midwifery mission work, we have provided free midwifery training and capacity-building in low-income, high-mortality countries as a service to local midwives working anywhere in the community. In addition to the Philippines, I have invested in midwives in many other countries, and continue to do so. I have personally taught maternal and child health for free to national midwives and healthcare workers in Laos, Thailand, Nepal, Cambodia, Hong Kong, and India. Beyond the Philippines, we currently support midwives working in Haiti, Madagascar, Mexico, Tanzania, Ethiopia, and Uganda.

In 2012, I was at my home in the Philippines hosting a midwife visiting from America. Michelle was of Philippine ancestry, and we were talking about birth outcomes around the world. I shared that I had known for over a decade that Black and Indigenous babies in America were dying at birth at least twice as often than white babies, a fact that made me extremely concerned, but I was living and working in the Philippines, not America, so I figured there was nothing I could personally do. Now we were discussing the new data that was showing a rate of maternal death that was also much higher among women identified as Black or Indigenous.

Suddenly, in the midst of our conversation, I had an epiphany: Maybe what we were doing in poor countries—targeted educational scholarships for midwives—could work in America, too, if our midwifery school strategically designed a scholarship to save lives. Free education wouldn't fix all the problems, of course, but it was a start toward training more midwives in communities with the most vulnerable populations.

That was the beginning of Mercy In Action's scholarship program to support midwife students from high-risk populations who are most likely to lose mothers and babies around the time of birth. At present, the highest death rates in the perinatal period in the United States are still seen in Black communities, followed by American Indian and Alaska Native communities, so these are the groups who currently qualify for our scholarship. As of this writing, Black mothers and their newborns face maternal and infant mortality rates that are three to four times higher than those seen among White, Hispanic, or Asian populations in America. While maternal and newborn mortality remain high overall in the United States compared to other wealthy nations, the disparity gap continues to widen.

Because we have a caring and generous group of individuals serving on Mercy In Action's board of directors, we did not wait to raise outside funds before launching the scholarship program. Mercy In Action's College of Midwifery has, as of this writing, awarded more than half a million US dollars in scholarships between 2012 and 2025, most of it drawn from our general budget. And because the crisis in maternity care remains urgent for Black and Indigenous communities, we are not limiting how many scholarships we award each year to qualified midwifery students. At our current pace, we expect to give away another half million dollars from our general budget within the next few years. We now also have a donation fund set up on GlobalGiving's site, so anyone can contribute to these scholarships if they desire to join this good cause.

In 2013 Jan Tritten published an article about our scholarship in *Midwifery Today*, and my friends Jennie Joseph and Claudia Booker, both Black midwives from the USA, wrote a postscript asking every midwifery school to do what Mercy In Action was doing in offering focused scholarships. Claudia, who later served as our scholarship coordinator until her death in 2020, wrote in her postscript, "When I received an e-mail about the Mercy In Action full scholarship program, I immediately wrote Vicki an e-mail entitled, 'My heart is singing.' Those are no small words for me. It was as if pieces of various midwives' and future midwives' dreams and the wishes of their respective hearts were being shared across this planet and were finding ways to make these dreams come true. Women of color in places too numerous to list had been praying 'for a way to be made clear'; midwives of conscience and an undying commitment to saving mothers and babies were scratching their heads and counting their pennies and asking 'for a way to be made clear.'"

That clear path opened the way for a young woman named Sumayya Sulaiman, who was awarded the scholarship in 2015. She excelled in our midwifery school and graduated with distinction, and later joined our fold as staff and faculty. Sumayya's warm heart and enthusiasm are contagious, and she embodies the vision behind this scholarship. When Claudia passed away, we named our Mercy In Action scholarship in her honor, and Sumayya took her place as our scholarship coordinator.

Naming the scholarship after Claudia meant so much to many recipients, including Jada Rush, who wrote this: "After my husband and I lost our third baby girl during labor, I could not even begin to imagine that I would ever resume my midwifery journey. It was then that I saw in a vision a running track and Claudia reaching back, handing me a baton. A baton to continue the race...legacy being passed from her hands to mine." Jada not only graduated from Mercy In Action College of Midwifery after receiving the scholarship; she is now on our teaching faculty, generously helping other students to succeed.

Another midwife graduate of our college who now works with us, Ashley Jungjohan, wrote this in answer to my question of what it meant to her to receive our scholarship: "It can be summarized in the phrase: to breathe and to be seen. In moments when the stress felt overwhelming, when burdens seemed crushing, and when the path ahead appeared impossible, this scholarship created space—a way forward, a place of rest, and room to breathe. It represented benevolent generosity rooted in vision and purpose long established before me. The financial support carried a deeper message: who you are matters, and the women who are dying—women who look like you—matter too."

My hope is that you too will look for ways to support the future midwives in your country, state, or province who identify with the people groups losing the most babies and mothers at birth. We called our scholarship a Grand Challenge because we were asking all midwifery schools to follow our lead in supporting future midwives from groups that are statistically more likely to lose their babies and mothers in childbirth. It's a start, and now you know about it, too. Perhaps you may be inspired to create a new scholarship or donate to existing scholarship funds to support future midwives who need it most.

DIPLOMA IN INTERNATIONAL MIDWIFERY & MATERNAL/CHILD HEALTH

When I first went to serve in low-resource countries decades ago, I quickly realized how much I did not know and how few practical resources existed to help me learn. I figured it out eventually, often the hard way, and thirty-some years later, I designed this course to fill that gap, offering the knowledge, tools, resources, and real-world guidance I would have given anything to have at the time I started on this journey.

Mercy In Action is committed to maternal and newborn survival everywhere in the world, and it is with this goal in mind that we offer this postgraduate midwifery diploma program. This is a multifaceted program like no other that exists today. Based on the belief that when maternal and newborn survival is the issue, skilled midwives are an evidence-based solution, this program allows scholars to learn from and partner in capacity building with midwives in low- to middle-income countries. One unique and invaluable aspect of the program is that students receive written feedback on their assignments from local midwives in countries with high mortality, such as those they are studying. Through the academic curriculum design, our diploma scholars are partnering with midwives globally to scale up best-practice maternity care. While learning, they are also giving back and honoring the midwives from other countries. This is an example of a strategy we use to educate, build capacity, and improve outcomes simultaneously.

Our diploma program teaches a global perspective, covers material beyond what is taught in initial midwifery education, and has the potential to save lives and make a lasting difference in the global maternity care crisis. The program is designed to be completed on a one-year track or a slower two-year track, with extensions available. The academic work is completed from a distance so students can continue their lives in birth work. Only one live event is required, and this in-person four-day workshop is offered on different continents each year, so it is accessible to our international students everywhere.

Enrollment in our Mercy In Action Diploma in International Midwifery program is open to midwives from any country, and the similar Diploma in International Maternal/Child Health is open to anyone who has finished high school and desires to help mothers and babies survive and thrive. No healthcare background is required for the diploma in maternal and child health. In both tracks, the heart of this diploma training is to enhance the work of midwives in low-resource and high-mortality countries.

SEMINARS AND ONLINE CONTINUING EDUCATION

For years, Mercy In Action has been a leader in providing continuing education for midwives. We have created dozens of online and live seminars and continue to develop more, on topics such as global midwifery skills, maternity care in low-resource settings, preventing mother-to-child transmission of deadly diseases, cultural competency, and respectful maternity care. We have developed courses with practical updated instructions for clinical practice, including IV therapy, suturing principles, pharmacology, and the use of the NASG. Because of our commitment to educational excellence, whether pre-service or in-service, we gladly expend the extra effort and expense to have our courses accredited and approved for continuing education credit. In this way our classes are a double help to midwives, doulas, and other birth workers who regularly renew licenses and certifications.

Continuing education courses and seminars are our way of giving back to the midwifery community, and they are another way we stay relevant, because continuing education, by definition, must include training that is new, current, and beyond basic pre-service topics. Midwives all over the world are required to keep up with their continuing education, so this is a wonderful opportunity to generously share with each other. Serving, teaching, and advocating for those with the least access to care, all with a desire to improve birth outcomes, makes it rewarding to continue to create new courses to share with birth workers around the world.

MY LEARNING JOURNEY

I am often asked how I learned the things I teach, so here are a few of the many continuing education resources I have used over the years for my personal and professional growth. These resources are available to learners in any country, are globally focused, and most of these programs are offered online.

The Global Health Learning Center

The Global Health Learning Center, now operated by the Frank Foundation, offers accessible, high-quality online courses for global health professionals. Originally developed by Johns Hopkins with USAID support, it has been an important resource in my own continuing education. Over the years, I have completed certificate courses in maternal health, child survival, neonatal health, and related areas that continue to inform my teaching and practice.

www.globalhealthlearning.org

The Institute for International Medicine

The Institute for International Medicine (INMED) has also played an important role in shaping my understanding of global health practice. Through conferences and online courses in areas such as disaster management and public health, INMED has offered training that bridges clinical care with real-world health realities. I have also had the privilege of attending and teaching at INMED's annual conferences, which are a wonderful place to learn and network with like-minded people.

www.inmed.us

Helping Mothers and Babies Survive

Most of our staff on both sides of the world are now certified as Master Trainers of these wonderful programs. We regularly offer workshops to teach Helping Mothers and Babies Survive topics as one part of our train-the-trainer workshops, and it is included in our Diploma in International Midwifery & Maternal/Child Health program. We have certified hundreds of midwives, doctors, nurses, and primary health-care providers in numerous countries who are now serving all over the world. We also welcome allied medical providers, doulas, and non-medical advocates into these trainings, because they are designed so that anyone with a heart to help can serve as a health educator. Every year, we move our training sessions to different continents.

www.hmbs.org

Wilderness First Responder

I have found my training in wilderness medicine and wilderness first aid to be infinitely helpful, especially in establishing a mindset for working outside of hospital settings. They train you to respond when no ambulance is coming and you have to utilize what is at hand, which is particularly useful if you will be serving in disaster zones or even rural maternity care deserts. This kind of preparation teaches a different way of thinking about assessment, decision-making, and the use of limited resources. For midwives, this training supports the ability to remain calm and decisive when conditions are challenging or rapidly deteriorating and medical backup is not immediately available.

www.nols.edu

Lead Like Jesus

Training through Lead Like Jesus has influenced how I think about leadership in midwifery and global service. I completed training to teach and facilitate both the Lead Like Jesus Encounter and the Way of the Carpenter workshops. These both emphasize servant leadership grounded in humility, character, and care for others. This approach has reinforced the importance of how we lead, not just what we do, and continues to shape the way I support leadership development among midwives working in diverse and demanding settings.

www.leadlikejesus.com

Coursera

I have earned many certificates over the years through Coursera, from universities including Yale, Harvard, the University of Pennsylvania, Emory, and the University of Edinburgh. These courses have covered topics such as community development, childbirth from a global perspective, quality maternal and newborn care, the science of learning, and positive psychology, to name just a few. I find the Coursera courses are concise and accessible while maintaining strong educational value. Overall, I appreciate having these courses available whenever I have a few moments to invest in ongoing, evidence-informed learning.

www.coursera.org

Central Seminary

In my sixty-fifth year, I completed a doctor of ministry degree through Central Seminary, a program designed to support experienced faith leaders serving in diverse and global contexts. The program emphasized integrating theological reflection with real-world servant leadership. For me, this training strengthened the inner formation I need to serve well in global midwifery leadership for the rest of my life, and it shaped how I can best support others in this work. The focus of my program was creative leadership, and my dissertation was on our First 1,000 Days program in the Philippines. It was a wonderful three years immersed in higher education.

www.cbts.edu

BOTH STUDENT AND TEACHER

There are many, many more sources I have used over the years to inform my life of service, including earning a second master's degree in intercultural studies in the Philippines after I earned my Master of Science in Midwifery degree in the United States. One of my favorite short courses I ever took was a hands-on week called Health, Culture, Agriculture, and Community, taught by ECHO Global Farms, led by missionary doctor Dan Fountain. This was a practical course for missionaries, Peace Corps volunteers, and anyone on the front lines serving the poor.

Over the decades, I have been greatly impacted by my good fortune to learn as I served alongside some fabulous organizations around the world. I took every opportunity to "pick the brains" of their leaders, gathering ideas and inspiration from people with great minds and big hearts. Sometimes those discussions occurred while hiking the steep foothills of the Himalayas or on a lunch break in Thailand;

sometimes elsewhere such as sitting on a beach, where a missionary doctor once described a procedure to me by drawing in the sand.

Another wonderful source of both learning and giving back for me has been presenting at conferences. These gatherings have been a meaningful part of my work over the years, allowing me to teach while also learning from fellow presenters. They have taken me from state conferences to larger international meetings, including teaching at the International Confederation of Midwives (ICM) Triennial Congress and ICM's Asia Pacific Region Congress. I have been a guest lecturer for University of the Nations many times and in several countries, where I meet the most fascinating people from all over the world. Each experience has shaped me both as a midwife and as a communicator.

During the COVID pandemic, I began teaching and consulting online, connecting with universities and hospitals in many parts of the world. What started as a necessity became an unexpected gift, opening doors to share across countries and cultures. Online conferences further expanded this reach, and during the lockdowns, I taught for the Microbirth conference in England, the International Federation of Gynecology and Obstetrics (FIGO) conference in Paris, and the Spinning Babies World Confluence. Online annual events like the Virtual International Day of the Midwife continue to allow me to share our model in meaningful ways, no matter where I am in the world.

All these speaking engagements have greatly enriched my life as a midwife, educator, and leader. As anyone who teaches knows, for every hour we teach, we spend at least triple that amount of time in preparing, and our own understanding is greatly enhanced by needing to master the material enough to effectively teach it to others. I find that each time I am asked to share with a wider audience, I am given another opportunity to grow in knowledge as well as in grace and humility.

BOOKS AS TEACHERS

Books have always been my teachers. It is no secret to anyone who knows me that I love books, and I revealed books as my earliest teachers in the preface. Books show us life from different perspectives, while so often engendering empathy and igniting our imaginations in ways nothing else can. I consider books to be like friends and teachers who I want to spend time with because they have so much to tell me.

The bookshelves in my apartments in both the Philippines and the United States are overflowing with books. I tend to agree with the quote attributed to Cicero, "A room without books is like a body without a soul," and I have stacks of books around me or in my satchel at all times. Indeed, I confess that I often add to my overfilled bookshelves on both sides of the world by bringing home new-to-me old books found in used bookstores, thrift shops, or Little Free Libraries. Even if I don't have time to read them right away, I keep long lists of books I want to someday check out at the library. Of course, this behavior dooms me to the existential crisis of all true book lovers—the knowledge that I will probably die with books I wanted to read still unread!

Despite my habit of book collection, I like being generous with my books. If you came to my house to visit, I would likely offer to send you home with a book I thought you might like. If you admired one on my shelf and commented that you have always wanted to read it, I will send you home with that book. So imagine the recommended book list I placed at the end of this chapter, as well as the selected references lists, as my way of sharing with you. Books have a way of finding us at just the right time, and good books lead to other good books, so choose one you have not yet read and see where it takes you.

WHERE WE GO FROM HERE

As we end this book, I want to remind you of the convictions that have shaped every chapter. In these pages I have shared what I have learned about serving with purpose, intentionally forming character, practicing hospitality, and leading with integrity. I have offered frameworks and innovations that grew out of real needs and that offer real solutions. I have written about creativity as something most of us carried naturally as children and may need to recover as adults by letting go of shyness and caution when flexible thinking is most needed. I have shown how generosity, when it empowers rather than displaces local capacity, can change outcomes across cultures in times of disaster and deep poverty. Together, these chapters point to a culture of mercy, compassion, and love that is effective and far-reaching. A true birth model that works.

The question that remains is where we go from here, once we close the last page of this book. The answer is not complicated, but it is demanding. We act. We apply what has taken root in us through these chapters, what our hearts and minds recognize to be true. As we invest in education and spiritual formation, we share what has shaped us with others who need it too. We work tirelessly to create birth models that work where we live and serve. We choose generosity that restores dignity and creates a fair start for every baby. We do whatever it takes to improve birth outcomes because it is the right thing to do and because precious lives may literally depend on us.

Changing birth culture toward better birth outcomes does not require perfection, but it does require commitment and follow-through. I watch the sunset and sunrise every chance I get, which is to say most days, and I am inspired by the thought from *Anne of Green Gables*, in which Anne says how nice it is to think that tomorrow is a new day with no mistakes in it yet! If we dare to try to change the culture around how birth is viewed, hoping to achieve more just outcomes, we must expect both successes and failures. I think all of us involved in this work need to find what Sir Walter Scott called "the soul to dare."

Real change in birth culture will come when a global community rises to support this work, sustaining birth workers, investing in the students who will become the next generation, and shaping a better beginning for women, children, and families everywhere. Whether you are just beginning with optimism or feeling disillusioned after years in the system, there is always space for hope. Change in birth culture depends on people like you, and it is not too late to deepen or rediscover your sense of purpose. You can begin now to shape a vision, mission, and strategy that improves outcomes and brings deeper meaning into your work.

I remember many times hearing Rose, in her role as a clinical preceptor, challenge the students she mentors to consider whether they want to be good midwives or truly great ones. This phrase carries two equally important meanings. First, it is a challenge to dig deeper, go the extra mile, and show greater attention, compassion, and generosity while keeping the needs of their clients above their own. Second, it is a challenge to be willing to receive instruction, accept correction, and remain humble. Great athletes rely on coaches throughout their careers, and great midwives think the same way, always welcoming guidance, feedback, and constructive criticism. Good versus great is a choice we make every day.

This is a timely reminder that midwives are uniquely positioned to walk among giants. The great ones live out their calling with a deep love for humanity and a sense of purpose that drives their service. Great midwives think differently. They give generously and act strategically to serve more effectively. With courage and grit, they tap into deep wells of creativity to continue serving, despite the harsh realities of navigating overwhelmed or broken maternity care systems. The great ones never give in to cynicism and never give up believing they can make a difference. As the Reverend Doctor Martin Luther King

Jr. so powerfully reminds us, "Everyone can be great because everyone can serve."

Personally, I am energized by training midwives and supporting safe and respectful maternity care clinics and birth centers because it is such important work. There is no higher calling than love, and we show love by welcoming the stranger, protecting the vulnerable, and spending ourselves on behalf of the needy. My granddaughter Zoe painted the words of the prophet Micah on three large canvases for our newest birth center to remind us: *Act Justly. Love Mercy. Walk Humbly with God.* I see these words every day when I walk into our clinic space; I feel them in my heart wherever I am.

Mentioning the paintings of my granddaughter reminded me of one last action for impact I want to leave you with. If at all possible, in as many ways as possible, take your family and close supportive friends with you on this journey. The road can get lonely, but traveling companions make all the difference. I have told in this book of how fortunate I was to get to serve side by side with my husband for forty-four years until his death. My role may have been more visible as the midwife who got credit for deliveries and guest-speaking, but ours was always an egalitarian undertaking.

At one time, four generations of our family lived in adjoining apartments in one large house in the Philippines. Now I live alone, but in the years since Scott died, my sons and all five of my grandchildren have come to visit me here, and each continues to contribute to the mission in different ways. My brother, cousins, nieces, and friends continue to show up for me with love and generosity. Surrounded by remarkable colleagues, I carry on this work, always looking outward to the good yet to be done, with no plans to retire.

I hope this book has made one thing crystal clear: Every one of us can help make birth safer and more respectful for those who are vulnerable. The responsibility to do so belongs to all of us. It will take a multitude of good souls from around the world working together.

Blessings as you go forth to find your unique role and part to play in midwifing mercy.

PAUSE FOR REFLECTION

Which areas of further learning within the field of maternal and child health excite you the most? In what ways do you want to continue to study the topics introduced in this book as you create a roadmap for your own continuing education? Start today by choosing one of the books from my recommended titles and see where it leads you.

RECOMMENDED READING

A SELECTION OF VICKI'S BOOKS ABOUT INSPIRING PEOPLE AND IDEAS

Appreciative Inquiry: A Positive Revolution in Change, by David Cooperrider.

The Artisan Soul: Crafting Your Life into a Work of Art, by Erwin Raphael McManus.

Attending Others: A Doctor's Education in Bodies and Words, by Brian Volck.

The Awakened Woman: Remembering & Reigniting Our Sacred Dreams, by Tererai Trent.

The Barbarian Way: Unleash the Untamed Faith Within, by Erwin Raphael McManus.

Better: A Surgeon's Notes on Performance, by Atul Gawande.

Birth Models That Work, by Robbie Davis-Floyd.

A Chance to Die: The Life and Legacy of Amy Carmichael, by Elisabeth Elliot.

Change by Design: How Design Thinking Transforms Organizations and Inspires Innovation, by Tim Brown.

Chasing the Dragon, by Jackie Pullinger.

The Checklist Manifesto: How to Get Things Right, by Atul Gawande.

The Children Who Sleep by the River, by Debbie Taylor.

The Creativity Choice: The Science of Making Decisions to Turn Ideas into Action, by Zorana Ivcevic Pringle.

Crucial Conversations: Tools for Talking When Stakes are High, by Patterson, Grenny, McMillan, and Switzler.

Cultural Intelligence: Improving Your CQ to Engage Our Multicultural World, by David A. Livermore.

Dare to Lead: Brave Work. Tough Conversations. Whole Hearts, by Brené Brown.

The Edge of Tomorrow, by Thomas Dooley.

Fearfully and Wonderfully: The Marvel of Bearing God's Image, by Paul Brand.

The First 1,000 Days: A Crucial Time for Mothers and Children—And the World, by Roger Thurow.

The Game Changers: True Stories About Saving Mothers and Babies in East Africa, by Jean Chamberlain Froese and Patricia Paddey.

Give: Charity and the Art of Living Generously, by Magnus MacFarlane-Barrow.

Grit: The Power of Passion and Perseverance, by Angela Duckworth.

Half the Church: Recapturing God's Global Vision for Women, by Carolyn Custis James.

Half the Sky: Turning Oppression into Opportunity for Women Worldwide, by Nicholas D. Kristof and Sheryl WuDunn.

The Hole in Our Gospel: What Does God Expect of Us? The Answer That Changed My Life and Might Just Change the World, by Richard Stearns.

The Hospital by the River: A Story of Hope, by Catherine Hamlin and John Little.

How Great Leaders Think: The Art of Reframing, by Lee G. Bolman.
I Guess I Haven't Learned That Yet: Discovering New Ways of Living When the Old Ways Stop Working, by Shauna Niequist.
Kissing the Face of God, by Dale Walker.
Lead Like Jesus Revisited: Lessons from the Greatest Leadership Role Model of All Time, by Ken Blanchard, Phil Hodges, and Phyllis Hendry.
Learning Humility: A Year of Searching for a Vanishing Virtue, by Richard Foster.
A More Beautiful Question: The Power of Inquiry to Spark Breakthrough Ideas, by Warren Berger.
Mountains Beyond Mountains: The Quest of Dr. Paul Farmer, a Man Who Would Cure the World, by Tracy Kidder.
No Cure for Being Human: (And Other Truths I Need to Hear), by Kate Bowler.
No Greater Love, by Mother Teresa.
Out of My Life and Thought, by Albert Schweitzer.
Paul Farmer: Servant to the Poor, by Jennie Weiss Block.
The Ragamuffin Gospel: Good News for the Bedraggled, Beat-Up, and Burnt Out, by Brennan Manning.
Sacred Habits: The Rise of the Creative Clergy, by Rev. Chad R. Abbott.
The Science of the Good Samaritan: Thinking Bigger About Loving Our Neighbors, by Emily Smith.
Start with Why: How Great Leaders Inspire Everyone to Take Action, by Simon Sinek.
Tattoos on the Heart: The Power of Boundless Compassion, by Gregory Boyle.
Their Name Is Today: Reclaiming Childhood in a Hostile World, by Johann Christoph Arnold.
Think Again: The Power of Knowing What You Don't Know, by Adam Grant.
Too Small to Ignore: Why the Least of These Matters Most, by Wess Stafford.
Unreasonable Hospitality: The Remarkable Power of Giving People More Than They Expect, by Will Guidara.
Walking with the Poor: Principles and Practices of Transformational Development, by Bryant L. Myers.
We Are All The Same: A Story of a Boy's Courage and a Mother's Love, by Jim Wooten.
Wide Neighborhoods: A Story of the Frontier Nursing Service, by Mary Breckinridge.
Wishful Thinking: A Seeker's ABC, by Frederick Buechner.
A Woman of Firsts: The True Story of the Midwife Who Built a Hospital and Changed the World, by Edna Adan Ismail.

SELECTED REFERENCES

INTRODUCTION

Werner, N. (2024). *Birth statistics 1995–2024*. [Unpublished internal report]. Mercy In Action College of Midwifery.

CHAPTER 1: BEGIN WITH WHY

Buechner, F. (1993). *Wishful thinking: A seeker's ABC*. HarperOne.

Damon, W. (2008). *The path to purpose: How young people find their calling in life*. Free Press.

Davis-Floyd, R., & Cheyney, M. (Eds.). (2019). *Birth in eight cultures*. Waveland Press.

De Volder, J. (2010). *The spirit of Father Damien: The leper priest—A saint for our times*. Ignatius Press.

Hawaii Public Television KHET-TV. (1992). *Simple courage: An historical portrait for the age of AIDS* [Video]. The Walter J. Brown Media Archives & Peabody Awards Collection at the University of Georgia, American Archive of Public Broadcasting. https://americanarchive.org/catalog/cpb-aacip-526-8p5v699b0f

International Confederation of Midwives. (2023). *Midwife-led birth centres in low- and middle-income countries*. [Webinar]. https://internationalmidwives.org/series/midwife-led-birthing-centres-in-low-and-middle-income-countries

International Confederation of Midwives, Jhpiego, UNFPA, UNICEF, WHO. (2025, April 15). *The midwifery accelerator: Expanding health care for women and newborns*. https://www.unfpa.org/publications/midwifery-accelerator-expanding-health-care-women-and-newborn

Joseph, J. (2020). There's something wrong here: African-American pregnant women and their babies are at greatest risk in the USA. In B.-A. Daviss & R. Davis-Floyd (Eds.) *Birthing models on the human rights frontier: Speaking truth to power* (pp. 131–134). Routledge. https://doi.org/10.4324/9781003088783

Nouwen, H. J. M., McNeill, D. P., & Morrison, D. A. (1982). *Compassion: A reflection on the Christian life*. Doubleday.

Penwell, I. (2009). Selah's beginnings. *Midwifery Today*, (89). https://www.midwiferytoday.com/mt-articles/selahs-beginnings

Penwell, V., Penwell, R., & Penwell, I. (n.d.). *Cultural competency and respectful maternity care* [Online course]. Mercy In Action College of Midwifery. https://www.mercycollegeofmidwifery.edu/cultural-competency-and-respectful-maternity-care

Penwell, V. (2010). A hidden tragedy: Birth as a human rights issue in developing countries. *Midwifery Today*, (94). https://www.midwiferytoday.com/mt-articles/a-hidden-tragedy

Schweitzer, A. (1935, December). Visit of Dr. Albert Schweitzer. *The Silcoatian, New Series*, (25), 781–786. https://cornerstoneboulder.org/wp-content/uploads/2024/03/Schweitzer-in-The-Silcoatian-w-Permissions.pdf

Sinek, S. (2011). *Start with why: How great leaders inspire everyone to take action*. Portfolio.

Stone, R. M. (2018). *Birthing hope: Giving fear to the light*. InterVarsity Press.

Teresa, M. (1975). *A gift for God: Prayers and meditations*. Harper & Row.

UNESCO. (2023, December). *Midwifery on the representative list of the intangible cultural heritage of humanity*. https://ich.unesco.org/en/RL/midwifery-knowledge-skills-and-practices-01968

UNFPA. (2025, April 7). *Every two minutes a woman dies in pregnancy and childbirth: Tackling a global maternal health crisis*. https://www.unfpa.org/news/every-two-minutes-woman-dies-pregnancy-and-childbirth-tackling-global-maternal-health-crisis

Veith, G. E., Jr. (2011). *God at work: Your Christian vocation in all of life*. Crossway.

Volck, B. (2016). *Attending others: A doctor's education in bodies and works*. Cascade Books.

World Health Organization. (2023, May 9). *Global progress in tackling maternal and newborn deaths stalls since 2015: UN*. https://www.who.int/news/item/09-05-2023-global-progress-in-tackling-maternal-and-newborn-deaths-stalls-since-2015--un

World Health Organization. (2025, April 7). *Maternal mortality*. https://www.who.int/news-room/fact-sheets/detail/maternal-mortality

World Health Organization. (2024). *Transitioning to midwifery models of care: Global position paper*. https://www.who.int/publications/i/item/9789240098268

WHO, HRP, UNICEF, UNFPA, Jhpiego (Eds). (2025). *Compendium on respectful maternal and newborn care*. World Health Organization. https://www.who.int/publications/i/item/9789240110939

WHO, UNICEF, UNFPA, World Bank Group, & UNDESA/Population Division. (2025, April). *Trends in maternal mortality 2000–2023: Estimates by WHO, UNICEF, UNFPA, World Bank Group and UNDESA/Population Division*. https://www.unfpa.org/publications/trends-maternal-mortality-2000-2023

CHAPTER 2: BECOMING THE GIFT WE OFFER

Bowler, K. (2021). *No cure for being human: (And other truths I need to hear)*. Random House.

Brooks, D. (2015). *The road to character*. Thorndike Press.

Covey, S. (2006). *The speed of trust: The one thing that changes everything*. Simon & Schuster.

Cunningham, D., Gauslin, D., & Lambert, S. (2020). *Values matter: Stories of the beliefs & values that shaped youth with a mission*. YWAM Publishing.

Duckworth, A. (2016). *Grit: The power of passion and perseverance*. Scribner.

Gardner, H. E., Csikszentmihalyi, M., & Damon, W. (2001). *Good work: When excellence and ethics meet*. Basic Books.

Grant, A. (2023). *Hidden potential: The science of achieving greater things*. Viking.

Karon, J. (2014). *Somewhere safe with somebody good*. G. P. Putnam's Sons.

Keller, H. (2016). *The story of my life*. Fingerprint! Publishing.

Lewis, C. S. (2001). *The Screwtape letters*. HarperOne.

Smith, H. W. (2000). *What matters most: The power of living your values*. Simon & Schuster.

CHAPTER 3: ABUNDANT HOSPITALITY

Abrams, A. (2022, March 2). *Jennie Joseph Wants to Fix the Black Maternal Mortality Crisis One Midwife at a Time.* Time. https://time.com/collections/women-of-the-year/6150545/jennie-joseph-2

Commonsense Childbirth. (n.d.). Welcome to Commonsense Childbirth. https://commonsensechildbirth.org

Crouch, A. (2008). *Culture making: Recovering our creative calling*. InterVarsity Press.

Guidara, W. (2022). *Unreasonable hospitality: The remarkable power of giving people more than they expect*. Optimism Press.

King, M. L., Jr. (1968, February 4). *The drum major instinct* [Sermon]. Austin Area Heritage Council, Atlanta, GA. https://mlkcelebration.com/mlk-the-man/famous-speeches/drum-major-instinct/

Luke 10:25–37 (New International Version, 2011)

Niequist, S. (2013). *Bread and wine: A love letter to life around the table with recipes*. Zondervan.

Northumbria Community. (2002). *Celtic daily prayer: Prayers and readings from the Northumbria Community*. HarperCollins.

One Day's Wages. (n.d.). *One Day's Wages*. https://onedayswages.org/

Penwell, V. (2011). Elizabeth Gilmore Remembered: Through the Eyes of a Friend. *Midwifery Today*, (100). https://www.midwiferytoday.com/mt-articles/elizabeth-gilmore-remembered/

Penwell, V., Penwell, R., & Penwell, I. (n.d.). *Cultural competency and respectful maternity care* [Online course]. Mercy In Action College of Midwifery. https://www.mercycollegeofmidwifery.edu/cultural-competency-and-respectful-maternity-care

Saint-Exupéry, A. (1943). *The little prince*. Harcourt.

Swinton, J. (2025, June 29). In pursuit of homefulness. *Plough Quarterly*, (44). https://www.plough.com/en/topics/life/health/in-pursuit-of-homefulness

World Health Organization. (1996). *Maternity waiting homes: A review of experiences* (WHO/RHT/MSM/96.21). World Health Organization. https://www.who.int/publications/i/item/WHO-RHT-MSM-96.21

CHAPTER 4: UPSIDE-DOWN LEADERSHIP

Babylonian Talmud, *Sanhedrin* 37a.

Blanchard, K. (2007). *The heart of a leader: Insights on the art of influence*. David C. Cook.

Blanchard, K., Hodges, P. & Hendry, P. (2016). *Lead like Jesus revisited: Lessons from the greatest leadership role model of all time*. Thomas Nelson.

Bolman, L. G., & Deal, T. E. (2001). *Leading with soul: An uncommon journey of spirit*. Jossey-Bass.

Bolman, L. G., & Deal, T. E. (2014). *How great leaders think: The art of reframing.* Jossey-Bass.

Boyatzis, R. E., & McKee, A. (2005). *Resonant leadership: Renewing yourself and connecting with others through mindfulness, hope, and compassion.* Harvard Business Review Press.

Brown, B. (2018). *Dare to lead: Brave work. Tough conversations. Whole hearts.* Random House.

Gandhi, M. (2020). *The story of my experiments with truth.* Fingerprint! Publishing.

George, B., & Sims, P. (2007). *True north: Discover your authentic leadership.* Jossey-Bass.

Gergen, D. (2022). *Hearts touched with fire: How great leaders are made.* Simon & Schuster.

Goleman, D., Boyatzis, R. E., McKee, A., & Finkelstein, S. (2015). *HBR's 10 must reads on emotional intelligence.* Harvard Business Review Press.

Goleman, D., & Cherniss, C. (2024). *Optimal: How to sustain personal and organizational excellence every day.* Harper Business.

Grenny, J., Patterson, K., Maxfield, D., McMillan, R., & Switzler, A. (2023). *Crucial influence: Leadership skills to create lasting behavior change* (3rd ed.). McGraw Hill.

Heifetz, R. A., Linsky, M., & Grashow, A. (2009). *The practice of adaptive leadership: Tools and tactics for changing your organization and the world.* Harvard Business Press.

International Confederation of Midwives. (2022, January 4). *Guide for midwifery leadership.* https://internationalmidwives.org/resources/guide-for-midwifery-leadership

Kelley, T., & Kelley, D. (2013). *Creative confidence: Unleashing the creative potential within us all.* Crown Business.

Lencioni, P. M. (2012). *The advantage: Why organizational health trumps everything else in business.* Jossey-Bass.

Livermore, D. (2024). *Leading with cultural intelligence: The real secret to success* (3rd ed.). AMACOM.

Mandela, N. (1994). *Long walk to freedom: The autobiography of Nelson Mandela.* Little, Brown and Company.

Matthew 23:11–12 (New International Version, 2011)

Mercy In Action College of Midwifery. (n.d.). Online Midwives & The First 1,000 Days. https://www.mercycollegeofmidwifery.edu/online-midwives-the-first-1000-days

Morsch, G., & Nelson, D. (2006). *The power of serving others: You can start where you are.* Dust Jacket Press.

Parks, S. D. (2005). *Leadership can be taught: A bold approach for a complex world.* Harvard Business Review Press.

Peck, M. S. (1978). *The road less traveled: A new psychology of love, traditional values and spiritual growth.* Simon & Schuster.

Rath, T., & Conchie, B. (2009). *Strengths based leadership: Great leaders, teams, and why people follow.* Gallup Press.

Roosevelt, T. (1910, April 23). *Citizenship in a republic* [Speech]. The American Presidency Project, UC Santa Barbara. https://www.presidency.ucsb.edu/documents/address-the-sorbonne-paris-france-citizenship-republic

Tutu, D. (2000). *No future without forgiveness.* Image.

Willink, J., & Babin, L. (2018). *The dichotomy of leadership: Balancing the challenges of extreme ownership to lead and win*. St. Martin's Press.

CHAPTER 5: MISSION-DRIVEN MODELS AND FRAMEWORKS

Cheyney, M., & Davis-Floyd, R. (2020). Birth and the big bad wolf: Biocultural evolution and human childbirth, part 2. *International Journal of Childbirth, 10*(2), 66–78. https://doi.org/10.1891/IJCBIRTH-D-19-00029

Combs Thorsen, V., Sundby, J., & Malata, A. (2012). Piecing together the maternal death puzzle through narratives: The three delays model revisited. *Plos One, 7*(12), e52090. https://doi.org/10.1371/journal.pone.0052090

Davis-Floyd, R. (2018). *Ways of knowing about birth: Mothers, midwives, medicine, & birth activism*. Waveland Press, Inc.

Davis-Floyd, R., Barclay, L., Daviss, B., & Tritten, J. (Eds.). (2009). *Birth models that work*. University of California Press.

Davis-Floyd, R., Pascali-Bonaro, D., Leslie, M. S., & Ponce de León, R. G. (2011). The international MotherBaby childbirth initiative: Working to create optimal maternity care worldwide. *International Journal of Childbirth, 1*(3):196–212. https://doi.org/10.1891/2156-5287.1.3.196

Davis-Floyd, R., & Penwell, V. (2022). Become an implementing partner of the International Childbirth Initiative: A model for safety and respect in childbirth that works in every setting, everywhere in the world. *Midwifery Today*, (142). https://www.midwiferytoday.com/mt-articles/become-an-implementing-partner-of-the-international-childbirth-initiative

Declercq, E. *Birth by the Numbers*. Birth by the Numbers. https://www.birthbythenumbers.org/

Foundation for Health Care Quality. (n.d.). *Smooth Transitions*. https://www.qualityhealth.org/smoothtransitions/

Harman, T. *Microbirth*. Microbirth. https://microbirth.com

Home Birth Summit Collaboration Task Force. (2020). *Best practice guidelines: Transfer from planned home birth to hospital*. Home Birth Summit. https://www.homebirthsummit.org/best-practice-transfer-guidelines

International Childbirth Initiative. (n.d.). *The initiative*. https://icichildbirth.org/initiative

International Childbirth Initiative. (n.d.). *Watch the 12 step webinar series* [Webinar]. https://icichildbirth.org/press/12webinars

International Confederation of Midwives (2018, October 14–19) *International Childbirth Initiative (ICI): 12 steps to safe and respectful maternity care* [Conference presentation]. XXII FIGO World Congress, Rio de Janeiro, Brazil.

International Federation of Gynecology and Obstetrics. (n.d.). *International childbirth initiative*. https://www.figo.org/what-we-do/figo-projects/international-childbirth-initiative

JHPIEGO. (2004). *Monitoring birth preparedness and complication readiness: Tools and indicators for maternal and newborn health*. Jhpiego.

Klein, S., Miller, S., & Thomson, F. (2021). *A Book For Midwives: Care For Pregnancy, Birth, And Women's health*. Hesperian Health Guides.

Lothian, J. A. (2020). Feature article—The international childbirth initiative: Twelve steps to safe and respectful MotherBaby-family maternity care. *The Journal of Perinatal Education, 29*(2), 69–71. https://doi.org/10.1891/J-PE-D-20-00012

Miller, S., Abalos, E., Chamillard, M., Ciapponi, A., Colaci, D., Comandé, D., Diaz, V., Geller, S., Hanson, C., Langer, A., Manuelli, V., Millar, K., Morhason-Bello, I., Castro, C. P., Pileggi, V. N., Robinson, N., Skaer, M., Souza, J. P., Vogel, J. P., & Althabe, F. (2016). Beyond too little, too late and too much, too soon: A pathway towards evidence-based, respectful maternity care worldwide. *The Lancet, 388*(10056), 2176–2192. https://doi.org/10.1016/S0140-6736(16)31472-6

Penwell, V. (n.d.). *Expect the unexpected: Psychology of birth emergencies*. [Online course]. Mercy In Action College of Midwifery. https://www.mercycollegeofmidwifery.edu/online-expect-the-unexpected-psychology-of-birth-emergencies

Penwell, V. (2016). How a checklist promotes human rights in childbirth: The International MotherBaby Childbirth Initiative. *Midwifery Today*, (119). https://www.midwiferytoday.com/mt-articles/human-rights-childbirth

Primary Maternity Care. (n.d.). *Step Up Together*. https://stepuptogether.com

Wheatley, M. J. (2002). *Turning to one another: Simple conversations to restore hope to the future*. Berrett-Koehler Publishers.

WHO, HRP, UNICEF, UNFPA, & Jhpiego (Eds). (2025). *Compendium on respectful maternal and newborn care*. World Health Organization. https://www.who.int/publications/i/item /9789240110939

World Health Organization, & United Nations Children's Fund (UNICEF). (2018). *Implementation guidance: Protecting, promoting and supporting breastfeeding in facilities providing maternity and newborn services: The revised Baby-friendly Hospital Initiative*. World Health Organization. https://iris.who.int/handle/10665/272943

CHAPTER 6: CREATIVE INNOVATIONS

Bandura, A. (1997). *Self-efficacy: The exercise of control*. Worth Publishers.

Changing the Face of Medicine. (2015, June 3). *Biography: Dr. Virginia Apgar*. https://www.nlm.nih.gov/exhibition/changing-the-face-of-medicine/physicians/biography_virginia_apgar.html

Ecclesiastes 1:9 (New International Version, 2011)

Einstein, A. (1954). *Ideas and opinions*. Crown Publishers.

Garvin, D. A. (2000). The U.S. Army's after action reviews: Seizing the chance to learn. In *Learning in action: A guide to putting the learning organization to work* (pp. 106–116). Harvard Business School Press.

Gawande, A. (2007). *Better: A surgeon's notes on performance*. Metropolitan Books.

Gawande, A. (2009). *The checklist manifesto: How to get things right*. Metropolitan Books.

Headquarters, U.S. Department of the Army (1993, September 30). *A leader's guide to after-action reviews* (TC 25-20). Homeland Security Digital Library. https://share.google/VJNvAvlW1G83UGWpF

Levitt, T. (1983). *The marketing imagination*. Free Press.

McManus, E. R. (2014). *The artisan soul: Crafting your life into a work of art*. HarperOne.

Mission-Centered Solutions, Inc. (2008). *The after action review*. https://fs-prod-nwcg.s3.us-gov-west-1.amazonaws.com/s3fs-public/2023-06/aar-mcs.pdf

Penwell, V. (2016). After action review: A guide for midwifery students and preceptors. *Midwifery Today*, (118). https://www.midwiferytoday.com/mt-articles/after-action-review

Phillips, A. (2018). *Post-birth scoring chart: Developing effective tools to decrease maternal mortality and morbidity in the postpartum period* [Unpublished master's thesis]. Bastyr University Department of Midwifery.

Pringle, Z. I. (2025). *The creativity choice: The science of making decisions to turn ideas into action*. PublicAffairs.

United States Agency for International Development. (2006, February). *After-action review technical guidance*. (PN-ADF-360). https://fs-prod-nwcg.s3.us-gov-west-1.amazonaws.com/s3fs-public/2023-06/usaid-aar-guide.pdf

CHAPTER 7: MINDSET IN MOTION

Buechner, F. (1993). *Wishful thinking: A seeker's ABC*. HarperOne.

Copeland, M. (2014). *Life in motion: An unlikely ballerina*. Touchstone.

Dahan, O., & Odent, M. (2023). Not just mechanical birthing bodies: Birthing consciousness and birth reflexes. *The Journal of Perinatal Education 32*(3), 149– 161. https://doi.org/10.1891/JPE-2022-0007

Davis, E. (2019). *Heart and Hands: A Midwife's Guide to Midwifery* (5th ed.). Ten Speed Press.

Dweck, C. S. (2007). *Mindset: The new psychology of success*. Ballantine Books.

James, W. (2017). *The Principles of Psychology* (Vols. 1–2). CreateSpace Independent Publishing Platform.

McLean, M. T. (2016). Microbiome and midwives: A look at culture. *Midwifery Today*, (120). https://www.midwiferytoday.com/mt-articles/the-microbiome-and-the-midwife

Penwell, V. (2018). Expect the unexpected. *Midwifery Today*, (128). https://www.midwiferytoday.com/mt-articles/expect-the-unexpected

Penwell, V. (2019). The disappearing second stage. *Midwifery Today*, (131). https://www.midwiferytoday.com/mt-articles/the-disappearing-second-stage

Penwell, V. (2021). Birth interventions: A double-edged sword. *Midwifery Today*, (140). https://www.midwiferytoday.com/mt-articles/birth-interventions-a-double-edged-sword

Penwell, V. (2024). The strength of midwifery—Evidence on two sides. *Midwifery Today*, (149). https://www.midwiferytoday.com/mt-articles/the-strength-of-midwifery-evidence-on-two-sides

World Health Organization. (2024). *Transitioning to midwifery models of care: Global posi-*

tion paper. https://www.who.int/publications/i/item/9789240098268

CHAPTER 8: SHAPING A STRONG START

Arnold, J. C. (2014). *Their name is today: Reclaiming childhood in a hostile world*. Plough Publishing House.

Bonaro, D. P., Arnold, J., & Ringel, M. (2014). *Nurturing beginnings: Guide to postpartum care for doulas and community outreach workers*. Debra Pascali-Bonaro.

Department of the Interior and Local Government. (n.d.). *Children's first 1,000 days coalition partnered with DILG to beat malnutrition, stunting*. https://web.archive.org/web/20231224211057/https://www.dilg.gov.ph/news/Childrens-First-1000-Days-Coalition-partnered-with-DILG-to-beat-malnutrition-stunting/NC-2023-1294

Fett, R. (2020). *Brain health from birth*. Franklin Fox.

Gradovski, M., Ødegaard, E. E., Rutanen, N., Sumsion, J., Mika, C., & White, E. J. (2019). *The first 1000 days of early childhood: Becoming*. Springer Nature.

Hanson, M., & Green, L. (2023). *What makes a person? Secrets of our first 1,000 days*. Cambridge University Press.

Hargis, A. (2018). *Baby's first year milestones: Promote & celebrate your baby's development with monthly games & activities*. Rockridge Press.

Karakochuk, C. D., Whitfield, K. C., Green, T. J., & Kraemer, K. (Eds.). (2017). *The biology of the first 1,000 days*. CRC Press.

Korczak, J. (2018). *How to love a child and other selected works* (Vol. 1) (Paloff, B., Trans.; Czernow. A., M. Ed.). Vallentine Mitchell. (Original work published 1919).

Landels, B. (2022) *Finding their feet: Every parent's guide to milestones and movement*. Bernie Landels.

Norman, A. (2019). *From conception to two years: Development, policy and practice*. Routledge.

Penwell, V. (n.d.). Mercy In Action and the First 1,000 Days. GlobalGiving. https://cl.globalgiving.org/pfil/56338/projdoc.pdf

Penwell, V. (2022). The role of the midwife in the first 1,000 days. *Midwifery Today*, (141). https://www.midwiferytoday.com/mt-articles/the-role-of-the-midwife-in-the-first-1000-days

Penwell, V. A. (2024). To survive and thrive: Nurturing the potential of every child through Mercy In Action's first 1,000 days program in the Philippines [Unpublished doctoral dissertation]. Central Baptist Theological Seminary.

Tharp, T. (2006). *The creative habit: Learn it and use it for life*. Simon & Schuster.

Thousand Days. (n.d.). *From cradle to career: The lifelong impact of early nutrition on minds and futures*. https://thousanddays.org/updates/from-cradle-to-career-the-lifelong-impact-of-early-nutrition-on-minds-and-futures

Thousand Days. (n.d.). *Why 1,000 days*. https://thousanddays.org/why-1000-days

Thurow, R. (2017). *The first 1,000 days: A crucial time for mothers and children—and the world*. PublicAffairs.

UNICEF. (2011, July) *Facts for life*. https://web.archive.org/web/20230619003102/https://www.unicef.org/reports/facts-for-life

Vanderpool, D. (2023). *Healthy moms → healthy babies → healthy communities.* Lulu.

CHAPTER 9: CROSSING BORDERS

American Academy of Pediatrics. (n.d.). *International Resources.* https://www.aap.org/en/aap-global/international-resources/?documentName=ECSB_Provider_Guide.pdf

American Academy of Pediatrics. (2021, November 15). *Essential care for small babies.* https://www.aap.org/en/aap-global/helping-babies-survive/our-programs/essential-care-for-small-babies

Bohren, M. A., Lorencatto, F., Coomarasamy, A., Althabe, F., Devall, A. J., Evans, C., Oladapo, O. T., Lissauer, D., Akter, S., Forbes, G., Thomas, E., Galadanci, H., Qureshi, Z., Fawcus, S., Hofmeyr, G. J., Al-Beity, F. A., Kasturiratne, A., Kumarendran, B., Mammoliti, K.-M., . . . Miller, S. (2021). *Formative research to design an implementation strategy for a postpartum hemorrhage initial response treatment bundle (E-MOTIVE): Study protocol. Reproductive Health, 18*(1), 149. https://doi.org/10.1186/s12978-021-01162-3

Boyle, G. (2011). *Tattoos on the heart: The power of boundless compassion.* Free Press.

Centers for Disease Control. (n.d.). *Group B strep disease.* https://www.cdc.gov/group-b-strep/?CDC_AAref_Val=https://www.cdc.gov/groupbstrep/guidelines/algorithms-tables.html

Centers for Disease Control. (2025, July 2). *Clinical overview of perinatal hepatitis B.* https://www.cdc.gov/hepatitis/hbv/perinatalxmtn.htm

Corbett, S., & Fikkert, B. (2014). *Helping without hurting in short-term missions: Leader's guide.* Moody Publishers.

Edmond, K. M., Zandoh, C., Quigley, M. A., Amenga-Etego, S., Owusu-Agyei, S., & Kirkwood, B. R. (2006). Delayed breastfeeding initiation increases risk of neonatal mortality. *Pediatrics, 117*(3), 380–386. https://publications.aap.org/pediatrics/article-abstract/117/3/e380/68616/Delayed-Breastfeeding-Initiation-Increases-Risk-of

Esegbona-Adeigbe, S. (2022). *Transcultural midwifery practice: Concepts, care and challenges.* Elsevier.

Fathalla, M. F. (2006). Human rights aspects of safe motherhood. *Best Practice & Research Clinical Obstetrics & Gynaecology, 20*(3), 409–419. https://doi.org/10.1016/j.bpobgyn.2005.11.004

Global Health Media Project. (n.d.). *Global Health Media Project.* https://globalhealthmedia.org/

Global Health Media. (n.d.). *Caring for yourself and your baby after birth.* https://globalhealthmedia.org/portfolio-items/caring-for-yourself-and-your-baby-after-birth

Gouvras, A. (2017, March 10). *Neglected tropical diseases and women; an International Women's Day special.* BugBitten. http://blogs.biomedcentral.com/bugbitten/2017/03/10/ntds-deworming-women-international-womens-day-special

Henderson, K. (2010). *Can fundal height be a good predictor of birth weight and identify low birth weight in neonates born to women of low socio-economic status in the Philippines?* [Unpublished bachelor's thesis]. National College of Midwifery.

Horst, T. S. (2017). *Dancing between cultures: Culturally intelligent coaching for missions and ministry*. Life Development Publishing.

International Childbirth Initiative. (n.d.). *International Childbirth Initiative*. https://ici childbirth.org

International Confederation of Midwives. (2024, September 19). *Essential competencies for midwifery practice*. https://internationalmidwives.org/resources/essential-compe tencies-for-midwifery-practice

Jourdain, G., Ngo-Giang-Huong, N., & Khamduang, W. (2019). Current progress in the prevention of mother-to-child transmission of hepatitis B and resulting clinical and programmatic implications. *Infection and Drug Resistance*, (12), 977–987. https://doi. org/10.2147/IDR.S171695

Kassebaum, N. J., Bertozzi-Villa, A., Coggeshall, M. S., Shackelford, K. A., Steiner, C., Heuton, K. R., Gonzalez-Medina, D., Barber, R., Huynh, C., Dicker, D., Templin, T., Wolock, T. M., Ozgoren, A. A., Abd-Allah, F., Abera, S. F., Abubakar, I., Achoki, T., Adelekan, A., Ademi, Z., . . . Lozano, R. (2014). Global, regional, and national levels and causes of maternal mortality during 1990–2013: A systematic analysis for the Global Burden of Disease study 2013. *The Lancet, 384*(9947), 980–1004. https://doi. org/10.1016/S0140-6736(14)60696-6

Lissauer, D., Cheshire, J., Dunlop, C., Taki, F., Wilson, A., Smith, J. M., Daniels, R., Kissoon, N., Malata, A., Chirwa, T., Lwesha, V. M., Mhango, C., Mhango, E., Makwenda, C., Banda, L., Munthali, L., Nambiar, B., Hussein, J., Williams, H. M., . . . Coomarasamy, A. (2020). Development of the FAST-M maternal sepsis bundle for use in low-resource settings: a modified Delphi process. *BJOG: An International Journal of Obstetrics and Gynaecology*, 127(3), 416–423. https://doi.org/10.1111/1471-0528. 16005

Livermore, D. (2009). *Cultural intelligence: Improving your CQ to engage our multicultural world*. Baker Academic.

Livermore, D. (2013). *Expand your borders: Discover ten cultural clusters*. Cultural Intelligence Center.

Livermore, D. (2013). *Serving with eyes wide open: Doing short-term missions with cultural intelligence*. Baker Books.

Livermore, D. (2019). *The curious traveler: See the world. Change your life*. Cultural Intelligence Center.

Livingstone, D. (1858). *Dr. Livingstone's Cambridge lectures*. Deighton, Bell, and Co.

Mandela, N. (1994). *Long walk to freedom: The autobiography of Nelson Mandela*. Little, Brown and Company.

Maternova. (2026). *Non-pneumatic anti shock garment (NASG)*. https://maternova.net/ products/nasg

Penwell, A. (2009). *Is the Birth Attendant a Risk Factor for Delayed Initiation of Breast-feeding and Non-exclusive Colostrum?* [Unpublished Master's dissertation]. National College of Midwifery.

Penwell, R. (2010). *Does a short interval between pregnancies cause low birth weight in subsequent babies born in the Philippines?* [Unpublished bachelor's thesis]. National College of Midwifery.

Penwell, V. (2018, February). Prenatal care in the context of a developing country. *Midwifery Today,* (124). https://www.midwiferytoday.com/mt-articles/prenatal-care-context-developing-country

Penwell, V. (2018, June). Labor and delivery care in the context of a developing country. *Midwifery Today,* (126). https://www.midwiferytoday.com/mt-articles/labor-and-delivery-care-in-the-context-of-a-developing-country

Penwell, V. (2019, December). Newborn care in the context of a developing country. *Midwifery Today,* (132). https://www.midwiferytoday.com/mt-articles/newborn-care-in-the-context-of-a-developing-country

Penwell, V. (2021, February). Postpartum care in the context of a developing country. *Midwifery Today,* (137). https://www.midwiferytoday.com/mt-articles/postpartum-care-in-the-context-of-a-developing-country

Penwell, V., Penwell, R., & Penwell, I. (n.d.). *Global midwifery skills: Maternal and newborn survival best practices* [Online course]. Mercy In Action College of Midwifery. https://www.mercycollegeofmidwifery.edu/global-midwifery-skills

Perez, K., Patterson, J., Hinshaw, J., Escobar, C., Parajon, D., Parajon, L., & Bose, C. (2018). Essential care for every baby: Improving compliance with newborn care practices in rural Nicaragua. *BMC Pregnancy and Childbirth, 18*, Article 371. https://doi.org/10.1186/s12884-018-2003-y

Ricalde, A. E., Velásquez-Meléndez, G., Tanaka, A. C., & de Siqueira, A. A. F. (1998). Mid-upper arm circumference in pregnant women and its relation to birth weight. *Revista de Saúde Pública, 32*(2), 112–117. https://doi.org/10.1590/s0034-89101998000200002

UNICEF. (2011, July). *Facts for life.* https://web.archive.org/web/20230619003102/https://www.unicef.org/reports/facts-for-life

Vitamin Angels. (n.d.). *Vitamin Angels.* https://vitaminangels.org

White Ribbon Alliance for Safe Motherhood. (2011, October). *Respectful maternity care: The universal right of childbearing women.* Harvard University. https://web.archive.org/web/20250720035618/https://content.sph.harvard.edu/wwwhsph/sites/2413/2014/05/Final_RMC_Charter.pdf

World Health Organization. (2008, February). *Regional consultation on nutrition and HIV/AIDS: Evidence, lessons and recommendations for action in South-East Asia.* https://www.who.int/publications/i/item/SEA-NUT-172

World Health Organization. (2008, September 10). *Hookworm-related anaemia among pregnant women: A systematic review.* https://www.who.int/publications/i/item/pntd-0000291

World Health Organization. (2013, June 30). *Consolidated guidelines on the use of antiretroviral drugs for treating and preventing HIV infection.* https://www.who.int/publications/i/item/9789241505727

CHAPTER 10: BUILDING CAPACITY AMID DISASTER AND POVERTY

Agarwal, P. K., & Bain, P. M. (2019). *Powerful teaching: Unleash the science of learning.* Jossey-Bass.

Alton, J. & Alton, A. (2015). *The ultimate survival medicine guide: Emergency preparedness for any disaster.* Skyhorse.

Coppola, D. (2020). *Introduction to international disaster management.* Butterworth-Heinemann.

Davis-Floyd, R., Lim, R., Penwell, V., & Ivry, T. (2021). Sustainable birth care in disaster zones and during pandemics: Low-tech, skilled touch. In K. Gutschow, R. Davis-Floyd, & B.-A. Daviss (Eds.), *Sustainable birth in disruptive times* (pp. 261–276). Springer. https://doi.org/10.1007/978-3-030-54775-2_18

Forsythe, A. (2013, April 16), *Fred Rogers: Look for the Helpers* [Video]. YouTube. https://www.youtube.com/watch?v=-LGHtc_D328&t=3s

Frank, A. (2002). *The Diary of a Young Girl* (B. M. Mooyart, Trans.). Bantam Books. (Original work published 1947).

Graham, T. (2014). *The genius of the poor.* Art Angel Printshop Commercial Quests, Inc.

Greer, P. (2015). *Mission drift: The unspoken crisis facing leaders, charities, and churches.* Bethany House Publishers.

Gutschow, K., Davis-Floyd, R., & Daviss, B. (Eds.). (2021). *Sustainable birth in disruptive times.* Springer.

Hill, G. J. (Ed.). (2020). *Relentless love: Living out integral mission to combat poverty, injustice and conflict.* Langham Global Library.

International Childbirth Initiative. (n.d.). *The initiative.* https://icichildbirth.org/initiative

Miller, D. (2015). *Rethinking social justice: Restoring biblical compassion.* YWAM Publishing.

Penwell, V. (2014, March). Mercy in Action midwives form disaster response to deadly super typhoon. *Midwifery Today*, (109). https://www.midwiferytoday.com/mt-articles/mercy-in-action-midwives

Penwell, V. (2014, September). Prematurity and kangaroo care during a disaster. *Midwifery Today*, (111). https://www.midwiferytoday.com/mt-articles/prematurity-and-kangaroo-care-during-a-disaster

Penwell, V. (2015, March). After the disaster: What comes next in the Philippines? *Midwifery Today*, (113). https://www.midwiferytoday.com/mt-articles/disaster-comes-next-philippines

Penwell, V. (2023). Buntis day party: A Mercy In Action imaginative prenatal model in the Philippines. *Midwifery Today*, (148). https://www.midwiferytoday.com/mt-articles/buntis-day-party-a-mercy-in-action-imaginative-prenatal-model-in-the-philippines

Penwell, V. (2023). Emerging strategies: Helping mothers survive bleeding after birth. *Midwifery Today*, (146). https://www.midwiferytoday.com/mt-articles/emerging-strategies-helping-mothers-survive-bleeding-after-birth/

Penwell, V., Penwell, R., & Penwell, I. (n.d.). *Midwives responding to disasters: Protecting survival in worst-case scenarios* [Online course]. Mercy In Action College of Midwifery. https://www.mercycollegeofmidwifery.edu/midwives-responding-to-disasters

Teresa, M. (2002). *No Greater Love* (B. Benenate, & J. Durepos, Eds.). New World Library.

Van Dyke, H. (2008). *The story of the other wise man*. CruGuru.

Veenema, T. G. (2018). *Disaster nursing and emergency preparedness* (4th ed.). Springer Publishing Company.

CHAPTER 11: ACTION FOR IMPACT

Alwy Al-beity, F. M., Baker, U., Kakoko, D., Hanson, C., & Pembe, A. B. (2022). Health workers' experiences of implementation of Helping Mothers Survive Bleeding after Birth training in Tanzania: A process evaluation using the i-PARIHS framework. *BMC Health Services Research*, 22, Article 1240. https://doi.org/10.1186/s12913-022-08605-y

American Academy of Pediatrics. (2022, July 15). *Helping babies survive*. https://www.aap.org/en/aap-global/helping-babies-survive

Angelou, M. (1993). *Wouldn't take nothing for my journey now*. Random House.

Bogren, M., Denovan, A., Kent, F., Berg, M., & Linden, K. (2021). Impact of the Helping Mothers Survive Bleeding after Birth learning programme on care provider skills and maternal health outcomes in low-income countries—An integrative review. *Women and Birth: Journal of the Australian College of Midwives, 34*(5), 425–434. https://doi.org/10.1016/j.wombi.2020.09.008

Davis-Floyd, R., Barclay, L., Daviss, B., & Tritten, J. (Eds.). (2009). *Birth models that work*. University of California Press.

Dweck, C. S. (2007). *Mindset: The new psychology of success*. Ballantine Books.

Ersdal, H. L., Singhal, N., Msemo, G., KC, A., Data, S., Moyo, N. T., Evans, C. L., Smith, J., Perlman, J. M., & Niermeyer, S. (2017). Successful implementation of Helping Babies Survive and Helping Mothers Survive programs—An Utstein formula for newborn and maternal survival. *PLOS ONE, 12*(6). https://doi.org/10.1371/journal.pone.0178073

Evans, C. L., Kamunya, R., & Tibaijuka, G. (2020). Using Helping Mothers Survive to improve intrapartum care. *Pediatrics, 146*(2), 218–222. https://doi.org/10.1542/peds.2020-016915M

Global Giving. (n.d.). *Claudia Booker Memorial Midwife Scholarship*. https://www.globalgiving.org/projects/claudia-booker-memorial-grandchallenge-scholarship/

Goffman, D., Joseph, N. T., Bhattarai, R., Knestrick, J. M., & Farinde, A. (2022, December 28). Novel approaches in the management of postpartum hemorrhage [Online course]. PRIME Education, LLC. https://primeinc.org/online/novel-approaches-management-postpartum-hemorrhage

Grant, A. (2023). *Think again: The power of knowing what you don't know*. Penguin Books.

Helping Mothers and Babies Survive. (2025). *Helping mothers and babies survive*. https://hmbs.org

Jhpiego. (2023). *Training and programming materials*. Helping Mothers Survive. https://hms.jhpiego.org/training-materials/index.html

Laerdal Global Health. (n.d.). *Laerdal Global Health*. https://laerdalglobalhealth.com

Keltner, D. (2023). *Awe: The new science of everyday wonder and how it can transform your life*. Penguin Press.

McManus, E. R. (2005). *The barbarian way: Unleash the untamed faith within*. Thomas Nelson.

Mercy In Action College of Midwifery. (n.d.). *Diploma in international midwifery and maternal/child health*. https://www.mercycollegeofmidwifery.edu/diploma-international-midwifery

Mercy In Action College of Midwifery. (n.d.). *Hands-on seminars*. https://www.mercycollegeofmidwifery.edu/hands-on-seminars

Mercy In Action College of Midwifery. (n.d.). *Online continuing education*. https://www.mercycollegeofmidwifery.edu/online-ceu

Montgomery, L. M. (1982). *Anne of Green Gables* (Collectors/Reissue ed.). Bantam Books.

Niequist, S. (2022). *I guess I haven't learned that yet: Discovering new ways of living when the old ways stop working*. Zondervan.

Oakley, B., Rogowsky, B., & Sejnowski, T. J. (2021). *Uncommon sense teaching: Practical insights in brain science to help students learn*. Tarcher.

Penwell, V. (2021). Future-thinking midwifery education: Birthing the midwives we need. *Midwifery Today*, (139). https://www.midwiferytoday.com/mt-articles/future-thinking-midwifery-education-birthing-the-midwives-we-need

Penwell, V. (2023). Mercy In Action—Still training global midwives after all these years! *Midwifery Today*, (147). https://www.midwiferytoday.com/mt-articles/mercy-in-action-still-training-global-midwives-after-all-these-years

Penwell, V. (2025, July 3). The midwife as student: Embracing lifelong learning. *National Association of Certified Professional Midwives Newsletter*. https://www.nacpm.org/news/june-2025-newsletter-education-frameworks-and-the-future-of-cpms

Penwell, V. (2023). The one-minute preceptor model for midwives. *Midwifery Today*, (145). https://www.midwiferytoday.com/mt-articles/the-one-minute-preceptor-model-for-midwives

Penwell, V., Penwell, R., & Penwell, I. (n.d.). *Navigating ethical student/preceptor/client relationships* [Online course]. Mercy In Action College of Midwifery. https://www.mercycollegeofmidwifery.edu/navigating-ethical-student-preceptor-client-relationships

Plueddemann, J. E. (2018). *Teaching across cultures: Contextualizing education for global mission*. IVP Academic.

Scott, W. (2020). *Marmion*. Biblioteca Press. (Original work published 1808).

ACKNOWLEDGMENTS

The world is a better place because of midwives who care enough to give their very best. To the midwives and midwifery students, past and present, who have served and studied with me over nearly fifty years, thank you. Together with my teams around the world, I acknowledge this book would not exist without the tens of thousands of women, babies, and families who entrusted us with their care. Patient names have been changed for privacy and respect throughout, but we remember each one of you fondly, and thank you for your trust in us at a vulnerable time in your life.

I am deeply grateful to the many people who helped bring this book to completion. Kristen Benoit, you were the first set of eyes on each chapter as it emerged; thank you for helping me juggle words and concepts to keep moving forward. Jenny Fox, you too read every word in real time and offered a constant voice of encouragement. Rose Penwell, thank you for pointing out what could be clarified and said better before we went to press. All of you helped me represent our model well. To all those who read early bits of my first drafts, Robbie Davis-Floyd, Michelle Skaer Therrien, Rachel Mast, Astrid Van Wingerden Guenthart, Michele Dondanville, André LaLonde, Carl Gilmore, Debra Pascali-Bonaro, Craig Allen, Zak Penwell, Anna Allen, thank you for your thoughtful feedback and engagement while the writing was still finding its way. Irie Penwell, I still smile thinking about you carrying that spiral-bound first draft from the Philippines across the world and sending me real-time photos from your phone of your circles around typos you found.

Thank you, Jamen Penwell, for spending part of your summer vacation at a desk in our Boise headquarters, surrounded by towering stacks of hundreds of my books, steadily typing up book lists by category and genre. Your cheerful endurance alone deserves recognition. And thank you to Keira Benoit, who spent many more hours at my table in the Philippines, bringing order to those book lists and reference notes with alphabetical and stylistic precision. Matt Benoit, thank you for stepping in with APA formatting expertise and other technical support. You are always willing no matter what I throw at you, and for that I am genuinely appreciative. Thank you, Selah Penwell, for using your college volunteer hours to gather research for my chapter on character. You gave me enough material to write two books! Thank you, Zoe Penwell, for your artistic help with promoting this book.

Marlene Domalaon, Nerissa Cumpio, and the Ponzio family, thank you for your courage and generosity in letting me share your sensitive stories. Thank you Neria family for sharing sweet memories of Ernie. Thank you to Jada Rush and Ashley Jungjohan for expressing how much our Grand Challenge scholarship meant to you; I only wish Claudia Booker were here to rejoice over your words. And thank you to everyone who sparked memories of stories, quotes, and anecdotes that helped this book show, not merely tell.

To my editors, Kristen Benoit, Ramona Denk Webb, and Joshua Glaser, you are the quiet wonder workers behind these pages. You corrected my spelling, rescued my punctuation, and untangled my sentences. This book is proof that good editors are both brilliant and kind, and I am beyond grateful. That you edited this from Papua New Guinea, Australia, India, Japan, and the Philippines only underscores that it has been a truly international labor of love.

To Ian Penwell, collaborating with you on this project was a dream come true. You never fail to make me laugh and make me feel cherished when we work together, especially at times when I need it the most. Thank you for the beautiful design of this book. Your unique blend of technical skill, creative genius, attention to detail, hard work, and vision shines on every page.

Jennie Joseph, thank you for honoring me and this work with your fabulous foreword. You are a kindred spirit; bless you always. And big thanks to all the busy midwives, doctors, and presidents who gave endorsements after reading an Advanced Reader Copy. I am heartened and humbled by your kind and generous words of advance praise for my book, Eugene Declercq, Neel Shah, Robbie Davis-Floyd, André Lalonde, Elizabeth Davis, Jamie J. Limjoco, Suellen Miller, Tigist Ejeta, Nicholas Comninellis, Roxanne Anderson, Pamela R. Durso, Debra Pascali-Bonaro, Jan Tritten, and Shafia Monroe.

And to the wide and often unseen Mercy In Action support network, our financial donors and monthly sponsors, grant funders, women's groups, churches, sewing circles, knitters, and providers of supplies, thank you. You keep this work going, standing behind us in ways that matter every single day. This book exists because of the merciful work you have made possible with your contributions and sacrifices. All the proceeds from sales of this book will go right back into the charity work that inspired it, and together we will continue to make birth safer and kinder around the world.

Gratitude feels too small a word for what I carry for each one of you mentioned here. This book may have my name on the cover, but it is filled with your fingerprints.

JOIN THE WORK

This work does not end with these pages. It lives in practice, in community, and in how we continue to show up for families and each other.

Learn with Mercy In Action

Our online courses are designed to support midwives with continuing education to bring this work into practice. These courses are available to anyone, anywhere, at any time.

www.mercycollegeofmidwifery.edu/online-ceu

Our seminars and workshops offer opportunities to deepen your learning, connect in community, and bring this work more fully into practice. Attend or inquire about hosting in your area.

www.mercycollegeofmidwifery.edu/hands-on-seminars

Our Diploma in International Midwifery and Maternal/Child Health offers a pathway to culturally grounded training that prepares birth workers to carry this work into diverse and resource-limited global settings.

www.mercycollegeofmidwifery.edu/diploma-international-midwifery

Prospective midwives in the United States can apply for our four-year Bachelor of Science through Mercy In Action College of Midwifery, which prepares students for skilled, compassionate midwifery practice rooted in this work.

https://www.mercycollegeofmidwifery.edu

Support the Work of Mercy In Action

As a US-based nonprofit organization, our work is sustained by the generosity of those who feel called to come alongside us. Donations may be made monthly or as a one-time gift, either online or by check. We also gratefully accept grants from donor-advised funds (DAFs) and gifts of appreciated stock. All gifts are deeply appreciated and tax-deductible to the extent allowed by law.

www.mercyinaction.com/donate

ABOUT THE AUTHOR

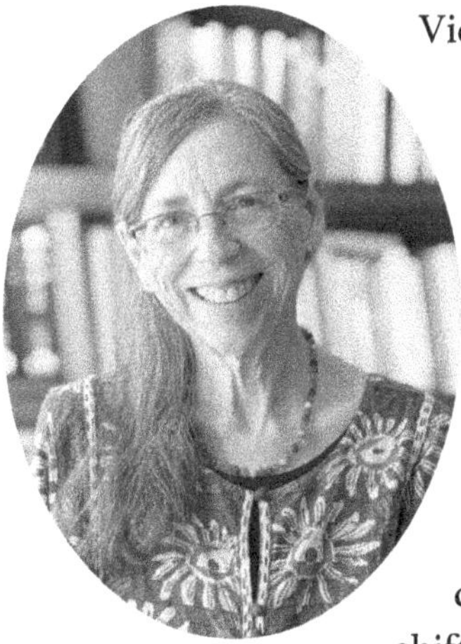

Vicki Penwell is a midwife, educator, and humanitarian who holds a doctorate in creative leadership and master's degrees in midwifery and intercultural studies. She is the founder of Mercy In Action Vineyard, Inc., a nonprofit organization that has provided free maternity care to thousands of families and has trained midwives worldwide. Throughout her career, Vicki has championed a paradigm shift in birth culture, challenging old assumptions and shaping new models of care rooted in mercy, service, and sacred purpose. Vicki is a frequent speaker and published author of over thirty-five journal and professional magazine articles, with additional contributions to books including *Birth Models That Work*, *Sustainable Birth in Disruptive Times*, and *Paths to Becoming a Midwife*. She divides her time between the Philippines and the United States, traveling globally to teach and mentor those shaping the future of birth culture.

Vicki can be found online at:

midwifingmercy.com

www.ingramcontent.com/pod-product-compliance
Lightning Source LLC
LaVergne TN
LVHW012039160826
845678LV00014B/2636

* 9 7 9 8 9 9 5 3 8 7 7 0 1 *